To Pippa.
In Friendship
from Lloyd
June 2001

Your Sort of Courage

Your Sort of Courage

Lloyd Kemp

The Lutterworth Press
Cambridge

The Lutterworth Press
PO Box 60
Cambridge
CB1 2NT

British Library Cataloguing in Publication Data:
A catalogue record is available from the British Library

ISBN 0 7188 2916

Printed in Great Britain by
The Cromwell Press

To the memory of Mary:

The mountaineer
In all his strength ...
Knows nothing
Of your sort of courage ...
As,
Scorning help,
With walking frame
And caliper
You move,
Step by step,
Precariously,
Alone in your weakness
Towards
The fireside chair.

Contents

Foreword

"You did look so funny when you were looking down at me!" That was Mary's comment several weeks later, once she had recovered some semblance of speech following her first stroke. We could think of nothing but what she had suffered. She had been lying on the landing floor all day, unable to move or respond to the insistent ringing of the telephone. Her only companion was Meg, a boisterous Welsh sheep-dog. Here, as always, her impish humour put all our anxieties into a proper perspective.

The title of this book is drawn from a line in Lloyd's poem *Slow Steps*, written to describe the heroic struggle of one person just to accomplish what is for others the simplest of tasks. Mary's courage, however, extended way beyond her own concerns. She was the mainstay of her family. As you read Lloyd's account, you will see how she was as much a support to him as he to her.

I have known Mary and Lloyd for a long time. Chance brought us together and thus I happened to be at hand at a particularly formative point on their spiritual journey. It was such a joy to find two people whose foundations were so strong that they could build new things upon them while affirming all that had gone before.

Theirs is a faith geared to bring consolation and strength to other people. Never triumphalist they have empowered their friends; at times cast down they have held their gaze on eternal truths. Living always in the NOW (or frantically seeking to do so!) their inspiration to others lies in the well-springs of their own experiences, even their pain. Lloyd's final poem in this book says it all:

"Each day a lifetime ... Each waking a birth ... Each morning a childhood ... High noon a middle age ... Each afternoon a retirement ... Each evening an old age ..."
> And night
> A return
> To the darkness
> Of unknowing."

To glimpse beyond that "unknowing" is to catch a sight of heavenly things. Sometimes some people may achieve this. I am sure that Mary's courage sprang from just such knowledge.

Tom New
Denbury, 1994

Bibliography

The following books are recommended for further reading – and grateful acknowledgement is made for kind permission from the publishers, and in the case of the books by HA Williams, from the author himself, to quote from these works.

Jung and the Christian Way, Christopher Bryant, Darton Longman & Todd, London, 1983

Collected Poems, 1909-1962, TS Elliot, Faber & Faber

Prayers of Hope, Richard Harries, BBC Books, London, 1975

Poems of Gerard Manley Hopkins, WH Gardiner, Oxford University Press

The Shaking of the Foundations, Paul Tillich, Pelican Books, London, 1962

The Eternal Now, Paul Tillich, SCM Press, London, 1963

The New Being, Paul Tillich, SCM Press, London, 1956

Friday Afternoon, Neville Ward, Epworth Press, London, 1976

Becoming What I Am, HA Williams, Community of the Resurrection, Darton, Longman & Todd, London, 1977

Tensions, HA Williams, Community of the Resurrection, Mitchell Beazley, London, 1976

True Resurrection, HA Williams, Community of the Resurrection, Mitchell Beazley, London, 1972

Acknowledgements

I wish to express my grateful thanks to my friend Hilde Auerbach, who read the manuscript as it was being written, and day by day gave me so much encouragement; and to many other friends – and particularly to Hilary Morrish – who, having read the newly-completed manuscript, were themselves so encouraging in their response. I also wish to express my gratitude to Patricia Scowen, Publications Editor of *Cruse*, who was instrumental in putting me in touch with The Lutterworth Press. I am also greatly indebted to Jenny McCall, Editorial Assistant at The Lutterworth Press, for her ever-helpful and always friendly comments and suggestions. Finally, these acknowledgements would not be complete without expressing my debt of gratitude to Harry Williams, without whose insights this book would probably never have been written.

Lloyd Kemp
Bath 1994

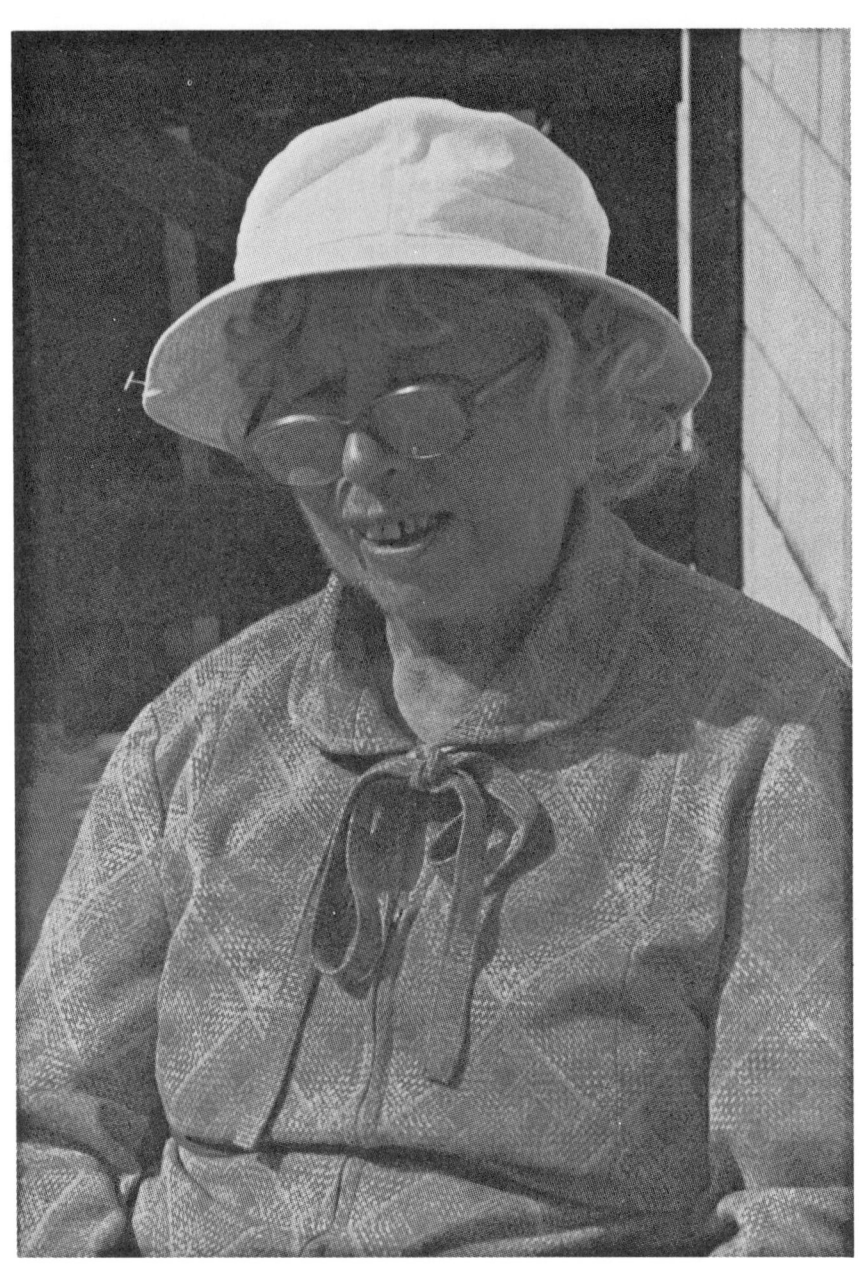

Mary in 1985

Chapter One

It was 7.30 on the morning of Monday June 17th, 1968, and even at that early hour the weather augured well, with only the merest wisp of high cloud, which offered no threat to the promise of a really warm day to follow. I have just scrolled back through my electronic calendar which, believe it or not, covers the years 1901 to 2099, to have it confirm my carved-in-stone memory that it was a Monday morning. As it scrolled back through those twenty years in its kaleidoscopic fashion, it also confirmed other searing facts burnt into the biochemics of my brain, for example that June 21st, 1977 was a Tuesday. But that began quite another chapter of Mary's story.

Mary had, as usual, followed me to the door, and stood watching and waving as I bounded up the steps of the little snicket which led to the next road and was my shortest route to the station. I looked back briefly and waved, and as I did so she turned into the house again – and closed the door on an era, though I had no inkling of it then.

In fact, as I jogged down the hill to the station, my mind was already stringing words together, which I would be writing down a little later, as I sped towards London. They would comprise the lines of a little poem – my vision of our new life together, in middle age, with the family launched and largely off our hands, and both of us with new work and interests looming for us to share with each other. The poem would be complete by the time I had reached work, and I would be so eager to ring up Mary, to share it with her.

Those were crowded days. Only two years before, I had left behind over 20 years in clinical radiation physics at The London Hospital to end my working days at the National Physical Laboratory on the more academic side. It was a big change at 52, and had kept me on my toes ever since. Meanwhile, our two sons had completed their university courses, the one in organic chemistry, and the other in architecture, and they had both married, whilst our daughter had left home for college, to study music. Mary, emerging from nearly thirty years of family life as wife, mother and housewife, had also blossomed – having just taken further A-levels to enable her to embark on a course at the local Polytechnic for the London University Extramural Diploma in Social Studies. She hoped to do case work in due course.

As I trotted down to the station that June morning in 1968 the sky, metaphorically as well as literally, seemed to be almost cloudless. The children were largely off our hands, Mary was embarking on an entirely new phase of her life, and my new work was full of fresh interest and challenge. As is so often the case when life takes on a new and satisfying shape, many a mountain was being reduced to a molehill and perspective over whole areas of our life together was being restored, revealing new vistas, and offering great promise for us both. Such were the prospects inspiring me that morning.

It was just after 9 o'clock when I made my first phone call home, clutching the single sheet of paper with the lines of the poem which I so much wanted to share with Mary, there and then.

There was no reply. Disappointment quickly bred a little chagrin. Why had Mary left home so early on this particular morning, of all mornings? Oh, I know! – she had been spending a lot of time in the Reference Library of late. But would the Library even be open as early as this? I put the phone down and busied myself with my in-tray. I would try again in half an hour. I worked my way through the tray, and picked the phone up again. Still no reply. Really, it was too bad. She would probably be out all the morning now.

Lunchtime came, and I still hadn't raised Mary on the phone. Reluctantly I wended my way to the canteen, had a quick lunch, and left my colleagues putting the world to rights as usual over their coffees, whilst I hurried back to my office, in the hope that Mary would have had her lunch out after a morning at the Library and would be back home again. The phone rang, and rang, and rang; and the length of time I left it ringing was a measure of the vague consternation which was growing within me. I had never known Mary absent herself like that without telling me of her intentions.

In the event I had to leave for home without having succeeded in contacting her, or having any idea of what had awaited her when she had turned back into the house that morning, and closed the door behind her.

The journey home, unlike the outward journey in the morning, was a completely fruitless one, with an irrepressible anxiety growing inside me all the time. It was vague and shapeless, and I tried to persuade myself that it was entirely without any reasonable foundation.

Why did I have to phone home from the station then, when I was only ten minutes away on the bus? I have no idea. But I did. And with the phone still silent, my worst fears began to take over. Clutching the poem in one hand, now neatly folded, with the inscription 'To Mary Mine, June 17th, 1968' on the outside, and my briefcase in the other hand, I took to my heels as I dismounted from the bus, and tore down the little pathway which led into our road, up the front steps of the house, and along the path to the side door. There, I found the morning's delivery of milk still on the doorstep. I knew then that tragedy, in some form or other, awaited me in the house.

I burst into the kitchen – the door was not locked – calling Mary's name as I went. I searched the ground floor – no Mary. I leapt up the stairs, two at a time. And there, on the landing, I found her – unconscious, in a pool of vomit. Later I was to be told that she had lain there since morning, where she had collapsed within minutes of my leaving.

Still clutched in my hand were those lines, written just for Mary, and which I had so desperately wanted to share with her all day. Snatches of them battered their way back into my consciousness as I knelt beside her: "*What does it matter, but that I love thee? ... meet with thee now ... finding each other, and ourselves, anew ... as the steaming mists clear, after the long day's heat ... early evening's cool refreshment renews the morning's promise ... free to love ... in time deprived ... of the tyranny of its passing.*"

I checked Mary's pulse. She was still alive and, as I gently lifted her head and eased a pillow under it and covered her with a blanket, I could only surmise that after I had left in the morning she had gone to make the bed and had succumbed to a stroke or a heart attack. She was to tell me many weeks later that all day she had been dimly aware of the phone bell ringing from time to time, and that it had been a strange, though remote, comfort to her.

I put what I felt to be the last and final fold in my vision for our future as I pushed it into my pocket and picked up the phone to ring the hospital, down the road and only half a mile away. On the assumption that the ambulance would come in a matter of minutes I rang Tom, our young vicar, and a stalwart friend if ever there were one. He arrived within five minutes and, stripping off his jacket, rolled up his sleeves and began cleaning up the vomit around Mary as I gently washed her face. We talked as we worked, trying to reach some understanding of what had happened, though deep inside me I was already desperately striving to persuade myself that it was only a matter of time before I came to and found that it had been just a cruel nightmare acting as some sort of counterbalance to the joy and optimism of my vision of that morning.

Despite Tom's presence beside me, I was hard back on my spiritual heels, asking what kind of early evening this was, which, far from renewing, had ended once and for all the morning's promise. What order of things could justify such an early end to such a vision? Tom was far too common-sensical to occupy himself with matters like that.

The minutes ticked by, and the landing floor was clean and sweet again, and there was nothing more to do but to keep vigil over Mary, and await the ambulance. A quarter of an hour went by, then half an hour, and I rang the hospital again, to be told that there had been some communication mix-up, but that the ambulance would be with us in a very few minutes now. Another half an hour, which only added to my general sense of unreality, but the bit of me that was still in the real world knew that it was prepared to wait no longer. I rang the ambulance service direct, and they were with us in ten minutes.

As they carried Mary out, one of the men, oozing a gentle air of superiority, offered the gratuitous opinion that she had had a heart attack. I didn't believe it myself, but assumed he had good grounds for saying so. He hadn't. She had, in fact, suffered a massive stroke.

The same night, and now in a full coma, Mary was moved to another, longer-stay hospital. The junior house doctor who had examined her offered me a second piece of gratuitous information under the auspices of the national health service – 'There's plenty of life in the old gal yet,' he said, assuming that if Mary had had a stroke she must be old. Actually, she was just 58, but he had entirely failed to register the fact.

They made up a bed for me in one of the side wards, so that I could continue my vigil through the night: no-one, at that juncture, was prepared to offer any sort of prognosis. How vividly I remember that night! A few minutes' doze, and then a tiptoe promenade along the ward, past Mary's bed. A little peep at her, and then on to the Sister's desk, to receive the latest comments, and a cup of tea and a biscuit. What a wonderful camaraderie it was, through the night hours! Years later I was to have the same experience all over again, and all over again was to learn that here in the small hours was to be found the quintessence of womankindliness. Despite the terrible circumstances which in a few brief, horrendous seconds on that June morning had destroyed all prospects for my vision of the future for Mary and me, the ward staff nevertheless managed to create a microcosmos within the narrow bounds of the ward's four walls, to which one felt privileged to belong. It was not simply that the barely tolerable pain of what had happened had been made just bearable, though that was achievement enough. Rather was it that in God alone knows what way they actually made me feel that this was the real world, the very essence of human life and relationships, of which the outside world was all too often but a pale reflection.

The morning dawned hot and sultry, and soon there was thunder in the air which, in a bizarre sort of way, seemed to match the cataclysmic nature of the events of the previous twenty-four hours. I stayed at the hospital all day until teatime, at which point a friend collected me in his car, in the middle of a blinding storm, and took me home for a brief respite from the long vigil. There had been no significant change in Mary, and I climbed into my friend's car in a stupor, like someone coming round from an anaesthetic; and I held out until I had just reached home. Then – despite the fact that a number of friends had foregathered to offer what support they could – the house, deprived of Mary, proved all too much, and for the first time the apparent calm was stripped from me. I broke down uncontrollably in front of the assembled company, the pent-up agony of the past thirty-six hours bursting the dam which I had tried to erect around it.

A woman colleague of the old ilk was shocked to the core, and remonstrated with me sternly. 'Don't cry, Lloyd,' she said, 'don't cry!' I suppose, since then, there has been some loosening of the 'stiff upper lip' convention for men, but there was at least one embarrassed person present as I wept my heart out in the middle of what felt like an apocalyptic thunderstorm.

Tom rang for news and, in response to my inevitable caution mixed with plain pessimism, he proffered the firm opinion that Mary was going to survive, and not only to survive, but largely to recover her powers again. Tom was certainly not in the prophetic line – he was renowned among his friends for his no-nonsense approach to life – so that his confidence in Mary's recovery was all the more encouraging. I knew he was the last person to indulge in idle soothsaying, which made me ponder the source of his reassuring words; but I didn't pursue the matter for very long, content to accept that there are more things wrought by prayer than this world dreams of, and that there are times when God does indeed move in a mysterious way.

The fact is that the next evening, just twenty-four hours after Tom's pronouncement, Mary opened her eyes for the first time, and her long march towards recovery had begun.

She had, among the other damage she had suffered, lost all power to formulate words. Her early attempts sounded more like what used to be called scat singing, or even (though I have never witnessed it) 'speaking with tongues'. At that stage, she never seemed to be frustrated by being completely incommunicado. The frustration came as she started to recover her speech. She had a totally paralysed right side, which meant that she couldn't write either, though later on she was to learn to write left-handed, in style.

It was I that felt the frustration. Time and again she would get so close to conveying her meaning, and time and again, with a little shrug, she would signify a philosophical 'Never mind'. Typically, a little later on, those two words were among the first she was to learn to say again.

Gradually, however, the incoherent burble began to take shape, only to lapse into a torrent of meaningless sounds again. How patiently she persevered – and how impatient I was, night after night, at visiting time, to detect the slightest improvement!

You saw me first tonight –
And waved!
And made a space for me,
A place for me,
Beside you,
On the bed.

Right from the start
We talked –
Oh, how we talked! –
You plainly,
So plainly, at first;
And after,
In that little burble
Interspersed
With laughter;
For tonight what matter
That meanings sometimes went astray
In wordless chatter?

What matter?
We met! –
Oh, how we met! –
In a fourth dimension –
Not of Einstein's time,
But freed
Of its constraint
And tension –
Where future
Had no past,
And past no future:
And the present moment,
Fleeting no longer,
Became
The Eternal Now –
The place
Of all
True meeting.

Mary's powers of speech continued to make steady progress, characterised, however, by frequent difficulties with some particular word or other.

'I can see the word' (she meant, in her mind's eye) 'but I can't say it,' she would complain, with real exasperation.

She was to say this over, and over, and over, during the next twenty years; and slowly, subtly, but steadily, the problem increased, as did her frustration. It was, indeed, the only one of all her problems (and there were many) over which she ever showed any such reaction. The reason is obvious to one who knew her. Mary had been a great communicator. In fact, life for her, ideally, had been one long state of communion with other people, who invariably stirred her interest, even though she might have met them only casually. She had a wonderful gift for making even near-strangers feel of real importance to her, and, invariably, they would leave her with the sense of their own significance enhanced.

Chapter Two

Slowly but surely, Mary began to gather strength, and to do what she was to do on so many occasions in the years that followed – continually to surprise, to confuse, and even to confound her doctors. During the early days of her illness I was repeatedly taken aside by them (understandably, I suppose, considering the seriousness of the stroke she had had) and told in sombre tone that I was not to expect too much, either sooner, or later. They had even hinted darkly that she might never leave hospital again, that she might have to be 'institutionalised' as they put it euphemistically. The notion was unbearable to me, even unthinkable, as I am sure it would have been to Mary, if they had ever dared to suggest it to her (ten years and two strokes later, I was to declare, in the face of what seemed equally fearful odds, that Mary was 'a survivor'). Even at that early stage, Mary's spirit had not yet been wearied to the point of exhaustion by years of handicap, and there was a certain natural womanly tenacity in her love for both her family and her friends (and such unfathomed depths to it) that it would never have occurred to her that the opportunity to express it again in the ordinary ways of life might not return. Her will to survive was something very special – it had little to do with the survival of her person as such, and much to do with the will of love itself to survive, her love for family and friends alike.

How magnetic that love became, in the years that followed! Those who started to visit her simply to keep her company in her largely housebound state found themselves drawn by it and by the warmth of it, not only for themselves, but for their families as well. She would ferret out all the details of children and grandchildren and the like, and would never forget them again; and immediately on arrival, on one of their regular visits, they would find themselves quizzed in detail, and by name, about each member of their family. Mary certainly had a badly damaged memory, but where it involved the material of her loving concern for other people, it remained razor-sharp. Surely there are implications here, for the largely materialistic approach of modern medicine, not only in the matter of the survival of that aspect of Mary's memory, but in the survival of Mary herself for so many years, and in the face of such terrible odds?

In those early days Mary had a good deal of so-called passive physiotherapy, but there came the time when they started to get her onto her feet again and, instead of bearing a war-weary, walking-wounded look, her face was more like that of a child learning to walk for the first time, with all its expression of anticipation and joy.

Once more, her uncomplicated responses were in sharp contrast to my own. I had been asked if she had a pair of strong shoes, with stout heels, that she was used to and that could be adapted to take a caliper for her right leg which, although gathering strength, still hardly belonged to her.

I retrieved her walking shoes from the depths of her wardrobe. How evocative clothes are, with all their associations, not only with their owner, but with the times and occasions on which they were worn! Twenty-three years on from that first stroke of Mary's, and three years after her death, the last generation of her clothes is still hanging in her wardrobe, and her outdoor coats in the cupboard in the hall. Morbid? If it were, I would have got rid of them long before this. I realise even as I write that there is a special reason why retaining them for so long is not morbid for me, and why they give me such a sense of Mary's closeness, even presence, still.

You see – I dressed her for those twenty years; she even entrusted to me the choosing and buying of most of her clothes. I seemed to have a gift for knowing what would please and suit her, and she was more than willing to be shot of the trouble of going to a shop, with all the business (especially for her) of trying out a dress in the fitting rooms. I had an understanding with a particular shop whose two middle-aged lady proprietors had a soft spot for me and were willing to let me bring home a dress which I thought would be suitable, for Mary to try; and so successful was I at this that I cannot recollect her ever turning down a single one of my choices! It certainly wasn't that she didn't bother much about what she wore; there was one delightful and memorable occasion when I brought home two dresses, for her to choose from, and she misunderstood, and said with great glee that she would have both of them!

As for her walking shoes, they had tramped such places as the mountains of North Wales, the Yorkshire moors, the cliff paths of the Channel Isles, and the Vienna Woods; and they would have taken Mary on a tour down the Rhine had the stroke not intervened and changed her life for ever. I could never quite get over their transformation from holiday wear to becoming the anchor for the steel pin of a caliper, giving some strength and purposefulness to a paralysed right leg.

Mary continued to play havoc with the prognostications of the doctors and, in little over two months after I had found her unconscious on the landing floor, she was discharged from the hospital. Frail, of course, and physically a shadow of the bustling self that had taken A-levels in French, History and Social Science only three months before; but if the bustle had gone and, alas, gone for ever, the determination which had enabled her to sail through three A-levels with good credits was undiminished. The difference was that instead of enabling her to tackle a brand-new subject like Social Science at 58, it was being applied to much more difficult tasks.

Slow steps
On familiar ground,
With carpet's edge
A dangerous ledge,
And single stair
A precipice,
Fraught
With grave peril:
The mountaineer
In all his strength,
Roped
To stalwart colleagues,
With the blue sky
And the towering peaks
Above
To challenge him,
Knows nothing
Of your sort of courage;
His risk
Seems small,
And his objective
Near,
Compared with yours,
A few feet away;
As,
Scorning help,
With walking frame
And caliper
You move,
Step by step,
Precariously,
Alone in your weakness
Towards
The fireside chair.

Mary's strength lay in the very *lightness* of her spirit. She just shrugged off the difficulties and setbacks, of which there were so many. Often, through the twenty years of trials and troubles which lay ahead of us, she would giggle her way through a crisis, actually anticipating my own anxious and fearful response and doing her best to dispel it before it had taken root.

There comes to mind an incident which in fact occurred three or four years later, when we were on some sort of relatively even keel again. Mary was able to cater for her own simple needs during the daytime while I was at work, with the occasional visit from neighbours to check that all was well.

In the middle of a busy morning, the phone rang in my office. I picked it up, with no thought that it would be Mary – she didn't often initiate a phone call, even in those days. Come to think of it, and bearing in mind how she was in later years, it is amazing now to think that she was able to dial a number then – especially in the particular circumstances in which she found herself that morning.

"It's me, Wiggles," she said ('Wiggles' was the affectionate nickname – of complex origin! – that I had given her many years before). "It's me, Wiggles." She gave one of her unique little giggles then. "You'll never guess what I've done," she went on. I prepared myself for a pleasurable and unanticipated anecdote in the middle of a busy, but somewhat boring, work spell.

Rising to the bait I said, "No, I bet I won't. Do go on."

"Well," she said, with another giggle, "I've fallen over in the hall and bumped my head on the wall, and I can't get up again, though I have managed to get to the phone. What do you think of that?" she asked triumphantly. The giggles were genuine and so typical, with not the slightest trace of hysteria about them.

I asked her about her head. "Well, it's got a bit of a bump on it, of course," she said, as casually as maybe.

I knew I wasn't going to get very far with her on that score, so I simply told her not to attempt any more crawling about, and to stay where she was, by the phone. I would ring friends who were only a few hundred yards away from the house and get them to go round. In the meantime, I would arrange to get home as fast as possible.

Just how literally true that turned out to be, I was soon to find out. I hadn't taken to the road to and from work as yet, and was still travelling courtesy of Southern Railway. To go home in my usual style and manner was out of the question – it would take at least an hour and a half in the middle of the day and I knew Mike, a younger colleague of mine, would be only too ready to help. He had come to know Mary well since her stroke, having visited us on a number of occasions, and was very fond of her. What was of more practical consequence at that moment was that he had a 5-litre open coupé American Mustang, which would go very fast indeed on the open road.

In a matter of minutes we had threaded our way through the urban traffic and were out on the A3, heading southwards. Most of it was a dangerous three-lane road, with the middle lane occupied briefly by the bravest (or the more foolhardy, as the case may be) for the purpose of overtaking. But there were also some stretches of dual-carriageway, which provided Mike with the opportunity of showing off the paces of his Mustang.

There was one never-to-be-forgotten moment along one such stretch as we were nearing our destination when, at over 90 miles an hour, we drove up to within five or six feet of the car ahead of us in the outer lane. There was room for him to pull over, and back into the inner lane, but he was as obstinate and as unyielding as Mike was at that moment – that is, until Mike resorted to his secret weapon. I wasn't aware of the existence of such a device, and probably the motorist ahead of us wasn't either. I've forgotten what Mike called it – 'alarm horn' will do for now.

Whatever it was, it emitted a piercing blast of sound which must have been up in the 110 decibel region at least. Perhaps the motorist in front of us thought it was some special sort of police siren – or even the Archangel Gabriel's trump! Whichever, he was in the instant back in the inner lane and Mike drove past him imperiously, at over 100 mph.

I read Mike the riot act then, and in particular told him in no uncertain terms that I would be of use to Mary only if I arrived home in one piece. We actually did the 25 miles in little over half an hour, including negotiating the urban traffic at either end of the journey.

We found Mary quite comfortable in an armchair, with our friends, and a lump on her head almost as big as a golf ball. I was appalled and, needless to say, immediately rang for the doctor.

He was relatively nonchalant about it and said that, anyway, there was little that could be done about the lump – it would disperse in due course and of its own accord – meanwhile, to keep Mary quiet.

She made an uneventful recovery, and went up yet another notch in Mike's respect and admiration.

In the sort of position in which Mary and I found ourselves after that first stroke, how one treasured the telephone – and the comfort and reassurance that it provides all the time, in such circumstances. Well, almost all the time; there was one terrifying lunch hour when it was quite otherwise.

As part of the daily routine once I was back at work, it was understood that I would make a brief lunchtime phone call home. It kept Mary in touch with me and enabled me to start the afternoon with an easy mind.

There came a fateful day when I got the ringing tone, but no reply. I had made the call from a call box while I was out walking after lunch. Fearing the very worst, yet clinging to what seemed a totally unjustifiable hope that there might yet be some innocent and simple explanation, I took to my heels and ran to the next call box, to try again. Still no response from Mary. I ran all the way back to my office then, feeling that it was a more reliable base from which to operate, compared with a phone box. Still no reply. I panicked and rang Tom, our vicar, ever and always reliable in time of difficulty or trouble. I hurriedly explained what had happened and asked him if he would go round and check up on Mary, and ring me back from the house. He was off like a shot, and in little over five minutes had rung back, to say that he had found Mary quietly having her lunch.

She told Tom that the phone had not rung at all – and yet he was actually using it to call me. I had a reassuring word with Mary, and then rang the Post Office.

"Oh, yes!" they said, "it is quite possible to get the ringing tone and yet for the phone not to be ringing."

"What sort of sense does that make?" I asked, furious over the implications of such a revelation for someone in my circumstances, needing a simple assurance that all was well at the other end of the line.

"You could have had the line checked," said the voice of officialdom, blandly.

"Why should it even occur to me to have the line checked, when I was getting the ringing tone?" I asked, still more furious at what seemed to me a particularly fatuous suggestion.

"Ah! well – " countered the voice, guardedly.

I rang off, and wrote to the GPO, and got a polite but totally unhelpful reply, to the effect that it was left to the engineer working on a line to decide whether or not to bother to switch on the 'Number Unobtainable' tone.

I wrote again, spelling out the consequences of such a procedure for the likes of Mary and me, and suggesting that they should change their ways.

Some 20 years later, I have just rung what is now British Telecom, and asked the same question: 'Is it true that if one gets the ringing tone, it doesn't mean necessarily that the number is ringing?'

"Yes, that's true," the voice said, with the same bland tone that the operator had used twenty years before.

All over again I spelled out the consequences for two people in the position that Mary and I had been in. Sadly, it was a hypothetical matter this time, for Mary had died three years ago.

The voice sought to escape via the usual route. "I'm afraid I'm not technical," it said, "but I could put you in touch with someone who is, who could explain it to you, I'm sure."

I'm sure he could, I thought. But I said, "Don't bother," and put the phone down. After all, if they haven't done anything about it in 20 years or more, nothing that I say now is likely to make any difference.

Chapter Three

The year wears on –
The magic mists appear,
Casting their immemorial spell;
And leaves,
Fresh green when you were well,
Are turning brown, then red,
And, twisting in the chill wind, fall
As dead –
Trees shedding
Their sad confetti.

Daily, the artist sun,
With prodigal palette,
Paints cosmic canvases;
And, night by night,
The stark stars,
Piercing the canopy of evening,
Stave off, still,
The gathering dark.

And birds, on branch and eave,
Incredulously yet sing,
To catch my spirit
Off-guard,
And evoke
The fierce pang
Of remembered joy –
Joy that I scarce now
Dare contemplate.

For as long as I can remember, I have had trouble with autumn – even in untroubled times. No "season of mists and mellow fruitfulness" for me to look forward to, as the days shorten. Of course I enjoy the colourfulness, as the dull, dark olive greens of late summer begin to acquire their first tinge of brown; the softness of the light too, even in the middle of day, and the gentleness presiding over the landscape, before the autumn gales sweep aside the last vestiges of summer. But there is a certain ambivalence about it. For all its beauty and quietness, the mood of autumn just below its surface seems sad, and heavy with a sense of impending decay. My friends used to try to take me in hand when real depression threatened, urging me to regard autumn merely as a forerunner of Spring. But I have never felt it to be as simple as that; autumn has always spoken of death as well as resurrection, and the one, in all its sombreness, must needs precede the other.

The effect of all this is to make me apprehensive of autumn, year by year, as it approaches; and when, in 1968, it coincided with the long haul of Mary's convalescence, and the growing awareness of the implications for the future of what had befallen her, it was doubly hard to bear.

There followed a long examination of the difference between happiness and joy, and the blessed discovery in the end that joy can, in fact, exist alongside great pain, a discovery eventually summed up in a postscript to the Autumn poem:

> Joy is no joy
> That needs to state its terms,
> And so deny its own true nature –
> Which
> Of such substance is,
> That neither time
> Nor chance,
> Nor circumstance
> Erodes –
> Or ever can.

The autumn had in fact come upon us by stealth, as we struggled to keep our heads above water in those early days of Mary's homecoming. Even the plans for the Rhine trip seemed to belong to another era, light years in the past now. Yet life went on for others, and one observed it with a strange sense of detachment, as though through a plate-glass window.

Friends and neighbours came and went, on holiday; and even the family, for whom life had frozen like a still from a movie film, got going again.

Our younger son and his wife stayed with us for a little while, on their way to a camping holiday in France, and it was their departure which after all these years I recollect as the moment when the full scale of Mary's tragedy was borne in upon me. It was the very first of so many partings which were to take place when members of the family, with whom we had shared a little of our time and a lot of our problems, left again, and left behind a sense of bereftness such as I had never before experienced. Moreover, faced with long stretches alone with Mary, and an ever-growing awareness of the terrible damage which the stroke had done to her, I began to experience the inevitable regrets, which slowly turned into self-recrimination and, finally and inexorably, into plain guilt.

Too easy it was,
By far,
To take you for granted
When you were well:
All too easy
To be preoccupied
With trivia –
To open the door
And peck you with a kiss
And say,
Straightway,
"Do you know
What so-and-so did
Today?"
Too easy
To but half-listen,
And never to stop
And wonder
At the music of your voice;
To let pass,
Unsung,
Your grace of movement,
The marvellous coordination
Of foot with foot,
Which we call
Walking –
Too easy,
All too easy,
So.

I mulled over the past, trying to discern the roots and origins of Mary's illness, inevitably, one way or another, starting to find reasons to blame myself. Gradually there came the glimmer of a vital truth – that all such exercises are at best sterile, and at worst positively destructive.

Years later I was to take comfort from the opening paragraph of a wonderfully wise book concerned with the suffering involved in failure, loss, and bereavement – the author Neville Ward, and the book, *Friday Afternoon*.

We never know fully what we are doing, what exactly is going on in what we are doing. The whole of the past is involved in every human situation. Most of it is infinitely diluted and untraceable. Some recent event is so clearly present that we are tempted to think it explains the bit of life it seems to dominate. However, we do not in fact understand. A hundred echoes from the distance, countless relations with the remote and the near, provide the clinging ambiguity that makes life so fascinating and at the same time so difficult to disentangle that it is obviously given only to God to see clearly why anything happens. (p.17)

Before Mary's illness, and in some other circumstance which might have provoked similar self-reappraisal, I would have been able to share my thoughts and feelings with Mary; but one of the greatest pains of that autumn of 1968 was the stark realization that I could do so no longer and that I would, indeed, never again be able to do so. Many weeks into her convalescence, Mary had at long last been able to read the poem which I had inscribed 'For Mary Mine, June 17th, 1968', but somehow it was borne in upon me that the damage left behind by the stroke prevented her from taking it to herself in the way she would have done had that June evening indeed fulfilled the morning's promise. That thought has remained with me ever since, a heartbreak which from time to time will always return to haunt me.

It is impossible to analyse, or even describe the subtle changes in Mary that the stroke had produced. One was inclined to attribute them simply to damage to some part of her brain. But even as I write these words I wonder whether suffering the stroke, coupled with her own inner awareness of what it had done to her physically, had not in fact caused her life to move into 'a new key', to borrow the musical metaphor which Neville Ward uses in a different context elsewhere in his book. Indeed, one may stretch the metaphor further, and say that perhaps Mary's life had modulated into a more remote, a more 'private' key, analogous to the keys sometimes reserved by great composers for expressing their deepest states of mind and spirit.

An even more profound thought comes to me now – that there was a sense in which Mary was, perhaps, already living in the world of pure spirit, the destiny of all of us, but which may have come to her twenty years before her physical death. Who knows? Indeed, who does know? The thought may seem far-fetched, even grossly sentimental or worse, but merely for it to have come to me just now is in fact a great comfort, imparting, as it seems, significance, even a solemnity, to what I had hitherto felt to be an impassable barrier between us and merely the brutal outcome of physical damage to Mary's brain.

Inevitably, I am reminded of what a bereavement counsellor whom I met on holiday once said to me some years before Mary's death, when I was describing to her this subtle sense of loss of close contact with Mary. She said, simply and straightforwardly, "It is a kind of bereavement, isn't it?", adding immediately, "I mean, a bereavement in slow motion."

Unbelievably, in early October, less than four months after Mary's stroke, we found ourselves at the Worm's Head, in the Gower Peninsula – *on holiday*. How it all came about, and how the doctors ever came to agree to it, I have no idea now; but it was typical of other, similar escapades which characterised the next twenty years. The 17th century French mystic, de Caussade, spoke of "finding one's only contentment in bearing the present moment", and it has seemed to me, as I look back, that Mary did find her contentment just there, *in* the present moment, or what Paul Tillich, the existential theologian, called "the Eternal Now". This gift of Mary's must have made all sorts of undertakings appear quite feasible at the time which now, with hindsight, seem incredibly hazardous. Thus, in 1969, we flew to Guernsey on holiday, and only a few weeks later to Germany, to our daughter's engagement celebrations with a young West German; and we returned there in 1972 and 1976. In retrospect, the motivation, and indeed the very courage to undertake such journeys, particularly those to Germany, can be seen to have come from Mary's all-pervasive involvement with other people, which almost totally precluded any concern or caution on her own behalf.

We had holidayed at the Gower three years earlier with my sister and her husband, and it was a 'play-safe' decision to return there – the last place we had holidayed at, and with which we felt, therefore, most familiar.

In the event it turned out to have been a grave mistake – I hadn't reckoned at all on the 'what-it-was-like-last-time' syndrome. On our previous visit, a change of job had been in the offing, Mary's plans for her return to serious studies had been well advanced, and we had seemed at the threshold of a new life in so many ways. It had been early summer too; and now it was well on into autumn – my sort of autumn, with the trees 'shedding their sad confetti', and being stripped daily more and more bare by near-gales off the sea.

We had a taxi all the way from Swansea, which put us down on the doorstep of the Worm's Head Hotel at the very beginning of the Worm's Head itself, and the terrain was such that Mary could not venture a single step off the hotel premises. Day after day I trekked the Downs for exercise, and day after day the contrast with our previous visit became more and more evident; and one of my autumn depressions of gigantic proportions set in.

It wasn't easy to assess what benefits Mary was getting out of it, either. The hotel was comfortable, and the proprietors very understanding and helpful but, so late in the year, we were the only guests, and even if our circumstances had been normal that fact alone would have made the place a little less than congenial. But, as things were for us, it all conspired to emphasise the drastic change that had come over our lives so suddenly, and how different it all was, compared with three years before.

My emotional immune system had not as yet developed the necessary antibodies against invasion by such negativities, but later on I was to learn the hard way not to wallow in a welter of 'if-onlys', and 'how-it-used-to-be's'. Again, I could not benefit from acquiring such antibodies from Mary, for the simple reason that she never, ever, got infected by such useless conditions in the first place.

The nostalgia all this evoked played havoc with my spirits:

> Menus on the tables,
> Places neatly laid –
> Sparkling glasses
> Waiting to be filled –
> Chairs disposed
> Invitingly;
> And, over all,
> The soft light
> Of the table lamps,
> Casting their benedictory air.
>
> I thought of the time –
> Oh, so little time ago! –
> When I took you out
> To dine:
> We sat in the sixteenth-century bay,
> Overhanging the busy street,
> As, Elizabethan-gay,
> We laughed,
> And ate,
> And studied the passers-by.
> And the toast was
> "To us!",
> As we raised the wine,
> And your right hand
> Held the glass –
> Oh, God! –
> Your right hand
> Held the glass.

Cynicism, and a sense of irony, invaded me too: no antibodies for them, either:

Pull up the chairs!
Poke up the fire!
And curl up,
Cosily!
For this week's
Colour Supplement
Invites us
To choose
Where we might go –
To escape
The winter
Within.

And let the chatter
Be loud enough
That the sound
Of the moan
In the wind
May be drowned.
Turn on the light!
Draw curtains tight!
(Yes! turn on
Sweet music, too)
And we'll play a game
Of make-pretend
That there is no darkness
Outside:
Better to bask
In fluorescent tube's light
Than risk
An encounter
With God,
In the night.

The Worm's Head was a mistake we did not repeat: never again did we return to an old haunt that we had known before the watershed of Mary's first stroke.

Chapter Four

Late that autumn we had the benefit of an informal second opinion from a specialist friend of mine from my London Hospital days. He had travelled down to visit us in our home, and had given us a guardedly optimistic prognosis to set against the routine cautiousness of the specialist who had been responsible for Mary at the acute stage of her illness. Because strokes were what happened to old people (or so, I think, went the reasoning behind the organization) Mary's 'case' had been dealt with by a specialist in geriatrics, and his opinion of Mary's chances was inevitably coloured by that. I am sure that he had made insufficient allowance for the fact that Mary was only 58 and, for that matter, that Mary was *Mary*. How could he? – he didn't know her: the advantage that our specialist friend had was that he did.

After all these years, I still don't know what the answer is, apart from having a doctor as a personal friend. What I do know is that I had to cope with the same partially sighted view of another specialist, in charge of Mary after she had had her second stroke, nine years later. He had been doing a ward round, and I was waiting outside the ward, until he had finished. He emerged at last, with his retinue of students deferentially strung out behind him, and spotted me as I hopped from one foot to the other with anxiety. He stopped in his tracks then, and came over.

"What your wife really needs is a new set of arteries," was all he could think to say, to comfort me.

What was expected by way of a reply to that? Again I don't know, but again I do know that there is something wrong somewhere, with a system which impersonalises communications to the point almost of dehumanizing them. There is no doubt that there are serious lacks in medical training – and in the approach to human *dis-ease* which this leads to – but I have more than a suspicion that the basic problem lies elsewhere: it takes time, a lot of time, to be human, and time is a commodity in short supply in the modern world.

Mary continued to suffer the vicissitudes of medical practice that winter. One of her drugs, only recently available, I believe, was a very sophisticated affair which was supposed automatically to regulate its effects on her blood pressure, according to whether she was sitting, standing, or lying down. So dramatic were its powers of adjustment (or over-adjustment) that we soon found out that there was a good chance that she would faint if she stood up too suddenly. Well do I remember one evening finding her flopped in a half-faint, and wedged between the loo and the loo wall (it was one of those little cubicle affairs). I could do nothing with her, and made an urgent phone call to the doctor.

To my dismay, so new was the drug that he arrived with the manufacturers' information leaflet at the ready in his hand, and proceeded to consult it as, together, we rescued Mary from 'her predicament.

She seemed to treat it all so philosophically, as though it was 'par for the course', so to say; and there is no doubt in my mind that it was for that very reason that she emerged relatively unscathed from many a tight corner.

We were well on into the autumn, and the 'second mile' of her convalescence, and I was beginning to be more and more aware of the changes which were taking place in my own life and daily routine.

"Bloody bad luck,"
He said,
As he drove from the fifteenth tee,
But it was not of his drive
That he spoke,
But of me.
(His ball went into the rough.)

  "Yes –
  His wife –
  It happened in June,
  And we've hardly seen him since;
  They despaired of her life
  At the time –
  Even now she can't be left."
  (They searched for the little white ball,
  Which, of course, was all in all –
  'Three off the tee'
  It would otherwise be.)
  "Damned bad luck –
  Just think –
  He's probably washing up!"
  (I was).
  "Poor bloody bod,
  Perhaps
  He's even
  Praying to God."
  (That also was true.)

They found the ball
(And another one, too),
And he chopped it out
With his Nine.
"We might save the hole,"
(His partner said)
"If the next one
Finds the green –
Yes, it's damned bad luck
When a chap has to chuck
His golf."

  By the time they had reached
  The Nineteenth,
  The washing-up was done,
  And my belov'd was up and dressed,
  And settled in her chair;
  And had started to practise
  To write her name
  With a hand that still rebelled,
  As they downed their beers,
  And swallowed their fears
  That life might not be
  Always
  A game.

Later still, that autumn, we learned that my sister had cancer. She went downhill with catastrophic rapidity, and died in a matter of weeks. There was another temporary lapse into near-cynicism then, in some lines penned on a lonely train journey to her funeral.

> Early morning
> Gives no warning
> Of a sunset
> Less than eternity away:
> No need to plan the day.
>
> Mid-morning
> Is refreshment time –
> Let's take a breather
> From our play
> (The sunshine has surely come to stay!)
>
> High noon,
> And native powers
> Intoxicate
> With the sense
> That the choice is ours:
> There is nothing we could not do
> If we wanted to –
> But we don't.
> By afternoon
> The shadow
> Of a doubt
> Appears:
> The sun seems not quite so high
> (Could it be that it threatens
> To set –
> And that in a finite time?)
>
> Late afternoon,
> And a nip in the air –
> Better to have a care –
> There is no doubt now
> That the night exists,
> And the light is getting low.
>
> But –
> Could it be
> That sun's dying glow
> Yet symbols
> A promise,
> Born of diminishment
> And fulfilled
> At day's end?

At last the spring came, and its limpid fresh greens lifted the residual pall of depression left behind by the autumn and its accomplice, winter. Mary was pressing on regardless, in her characteristic fashion, walking stably and safely now, with the aid of her caliper and walking frame; so much so that we had settled into something like a quiet routine again. We had organised a daily help for Mary (Julie, who was also a personal friend) who came in from mid-morning to late afternoon, did a little housework, had lunch with Mary, and generally kept her company. It meant that I could go to work with an easy mind, no longer haunted by the spectre of that day, the previous June, when there had been no-one to discover that Mary had been taken ill.

It was Julie who rang me up, in the middle of one afternoon.

"Mary has a bad pain," she said. "It came on after lunch. In her chest, she says. I've rung the doctor's. They'll let him know as soon as they can – he's out on another emergency call at the moment."

At that time I didn't yet have Mike as a colleague, so there was no Mustang to whisk me home in half an hour. Anyway, Mary was in Julie's safe hands, who, I was sure, would do all the right things.

So this time it was a taxi to the station, the first train I could get home, and then another taxi.

As we turned the corner into our little steep cul-de-sac, I was greeted by the sight of an ambulance outside our house, at the top of the road. The sight of it, and its exact position is stored like a photograph, in my mind's eye still. It is as though the impact of an event of sufficient moment acts like the fixative in the photographic process, preserving against further change the image of your world as it was for you, at that instant. How many such images were to be filed away in the photographic album of my mind, in the next twenty years!

Frantically, I paid off the driver, and rushed into the house. The doctor was there with Mary, who was obviously in great pain. As the ambulance men carried her out the doctor told me that Mary had a pulmonary embolism. I knew only too well the dangers of that.

Three hours later, when I went into the ward again after they had carried out a number of investigations including X-rays, Mary was sitting up in bed looking as if nothing had happened, and clearly free of her pain. Another one of those mind's-eye photographs stowed itself away then. As I scrutinise it, I can still see that expression on her face which I was to see on a number of occasions in the years to come. It almost baffles the attempt to describe it in words. There was a quiet and deep joy there, but tinged with a touch of fun, even mischief, which seemed to be saying something like, 'I wriggled my way out of that one, too, didn't I? – that caught you out, didn't it?'

It was the doctor she had caught out. His diagnosis had been very wide of the mark: Mary had gallstones.

More anxious weeks, eight of them, as we waited for the operation.

Our house was semidetached, and I cut a way through the tall dividing hedge at the back so that our neighbour could get to Mary quickly, should she knock the wall to indicate that she was having another attack. It never came, and she sailed through the operation.

Four months later we flew with friends to Guernsey for a holiday, and just a few weeks after that, to Germany, to those engagement celebrations of our daughter's. It all seems like a fairy tale now.

In fact, one could say that our long-range mobility at that time had far outstripped its more parochial counterpart. Apart from a spell just after the war, we had always lived in the country and, each member of the family being well equipped with two good feet and legs, and all of us enjoying country walks as we did, we had never felt the urge for a car. In any case, over the greater part of that period we could have ill afforded one; so that I had never learned to drive, and never had any great desire to do so. In these days, when two families in every three have at least one car, and almost every youngster hopes for driving lessons as a 17th birthday present, things are different (though not necessarily better). So much is taken for granted, and as a result so many of the joys of anticipation go by the board. If we had already had a car, of course it would have been handy from the start – more than handy. But the seriousness of purpose in learning to drive so that a whole new dimension could be added to Mary's life – well! – that was quite something!

I did actually enjoy learning to drive late in life and, in my advanced years now, I can still remember the thrill, comparable with that of Mr Toad himself, which I felt when, for the first time, with no-one else in the car, I drove through all the traffic in the centre of the town. It does make me wonder how many of today's youngsters will enjoy such a recollection in their late seventies...

I did very much enjoy, too, being Mary's chauffeur for all those years. She often used to say, as she sat beside me in the car, "You're a good driver, you know," but in the nature of things that couldn't be taken as any sort of a realistic assessment of my driving skills: it was, I am sure, merely her way of saying that she was happy to be out for a ride, and perhaps, as well, that she felt safe with me. Come to think of it, in those terms it probably did represent a judgement on my driving – it may even have been a sort of compliment after all – based on pragmatism!

Perhaps another advantage of learning to drive late in life was that I was aware, to the full and proper extent, that a car is a ton of lethal weapon; over the twenty years that I was driving, I never lost that proper awareness. However, when Mary had died, and the imperative for being on the road in a car was removed, I suddenly became aware of the jungle that modern traffic comprises and the jungle warfare that so often goes on there, and that 'proper' awareness quickly became an untoward one, so that I began to feel anxious and apprehensive all the time I was on the road. I gave up driving then: the motor car had served its vital purpose in our lives. I had never had more than a slight brush with any other vehicle, and by giving up driving when I did I shall be able to look back on that period of our lives and feel that the blessing that the car had been to us had never become a blight to any one else.

I sold B 164 WOU privately, and as its new owner climbed in, for the first time the car seemed to acquire a personality, and I felt I was losing a friend. I looked at the seemingly empty passenger seat in the front. In my mind's eye I could see, so plainly, Mary there still.

There was another thing I had to learn to do when Mary became handicapped, which I came to love and which, unlike the car, I have had no urge whatsoever to give up. It was cooking.

Mary loved her food. In spite of all her other problems rarely did she suffer any digestive ones. We had always eaten 'sensibly' (as they say), so that I didn't even have to make any special allowances for the fact that her gall bladder was no longer with her.

Prior to June 1968 my culinary skills, whilst extending beyond the proverbial boiled egg, were confined to such modest activities as frying bacon, making a Welsh Rarebit, and helping to prepare the vegetables for Sunday lunch; and in the earlier weeks and months of Mary's convalescence there was always Julie, our friend, to help out. Inevitably, however, the time came when necessity had to be the mother, if not of culinary invention, then at least of a slow but steady enlargement of my repertoire.

It all began modestly enough, but I am sure that my rapid espousal of cooking as a major interest had something to do with the fact that as a scientist the kitchen became a second laboratory for me. After all, cooking can be described in terms of measuring and weighing quantities of various substances, mixing them together in prescribed ways, and then as often as not heating the concoction at a carefully controlled temperature for a predetermined time. Put like that, it could just as well be a description of what goes on in many a well-managed research laboratory.

My modest beginning was with so-called flapjacks, which the dictionary describes as 'a chewy biscuit made with oats', which could indicate a quite sophisticated affair. But the recipe makes it all too plain that the actual skill involved is absolutely minuscule. Still, it was a start, and like almost everything else I made Mary not only ate it but gave it generous approval as well. As far as Mary's skills were concerned, there were more than a few in her nature that were quite untouched by the stroke, and among them was her capacity to encourage and inspire one in any fresh undertaking, ranging from embarking on an entirely different career within a year or two of our marriage, to making the humble flapjack.

I took to cooking like a fish to water, and I had soon added bread-making to my prowess at flapjacks. In the true tradition of the baker, I got into the habit of rising early (on a Saturday morning, when I didn't have to go to work), and the time when the loaves came out of the oven to fill the house with that wonderful and unique aroma of fresh-cooked bread, can be pinpointed by the fact that it coincided with the arrival of the weekend joint, delivered by the butcher's daughter who, like Mary, relished her food. I can see her so plainly (another of those mind's eye photographs) as she pushed open the kitchen door and sniffed the air approvingly, and with a delight which had its origins in a good appetite.

It must be said that cooking was far more to me than merely a congenial substitute for my laboratory activities. It was, and still is, truly sacramental, and I think it was understood as such between Mary and me. Indeed, although that part of our life together which preceded her illnesses is so long ago as to seem like another dispensation altogether (and a very hazy one at that, hardly belonging to me now), nevertheless one of the few clear impressions I retain from that time is of Mary's ministrations to the family having that self-same quality. Indeed, I must have acquired it from her in the first place. So, planning and preparing a meal to be shared with family or friends was (and still is) a celebration of the bonds of family or friendship, as the case may be.

But, once more, it is all a question of time, in these days of hurry and flurry – and of convenience foods.

Chapter Five

During that first year following Mary's return home from hospital, we were beginning to forge a new life for ourselves, saying goodbye forever to the old one and to that possible new one of which I had had such an agonising glimpse in my little poem. The backdrop of our new life would be the daily routine we would have to put together to accommodate our dramatically changed circumstances. My work still had to provide our 'bread and butter', and Mary's safety and well-being in the home had to be ensured. It is amazing how adaptable we all are under the harsh imperative of necessity, and looking back on those early weeks and months it is astonishing how quickly we – and most especially Mary – came to accept the enforced changes.

Our friend Julie's help was vital at that time, but Mary's ability to move about the house in safety and unaided steadily improved, until she could once again cater for her own modest needs during the day, and Julie's visits were confined to sweeping and cleaning and other household tasks which Mary would never again be able to manage. As for me, the whole experience of that first year redressed the balance in no uncertain manner, and differential equations took their proper and modest place alongside the equations to which life itself was requiring us to find solutions so rapidly.

Despite the many and obvious reservations which must be made about the motor car, there is no doubt that possessing one, and acquiring a licence to drive it, added a vital new dimension to our much restricted lives. Apart from enabling us to haunt the lovely Surrey lanes spread over the countryside for miles around our home, the car, once a year, did come into its own in a special way – enabling us to take a holiday which would have been unthinkable without it. Looking back from the vantage point of 23 years on, the distances we travelled, the risks we took (as they appear now, but not, strangely enough, then) and the relative remoteness of the places we visited, are well nigh unbelievable – from the Fens to Exmoor and Cornwall and thence (by helicopter) to the Scilly Isles; from mid-Wales and the Wye Valley to the rolling downs of Kent.

Well nigh unbelievable, yes, even foolhardy, those holidays seem now – but why? Is it because the shades of the prison-house have closed in yet again? Having lost Mary, and my role in life of looking after her, am I in danger of losing the art of living in the 'Eternal Now' which Mary was so good at? As I think about it, I realise that it was that capacity of hers which did indeed make all such adventures seem as safe as Sunday School outings though, alas, with not the same carefree and happy memories.

Holidays, in retrospect, usually appear as oases of fun and light-heartedness set in the relative desert of the daily routines associated with the rest of the year; and a mere mention of any particular holiday will invariably produce a rich fund of cherished anecdotes – already part of the family mythology. Not so those holidays with Mary. It is true that there were certain obvious practical advantages in being away, and staying at a hotel: no cooking, no housework, no shopping, for example. But living away from our home base we were to a large extent deprived of the routines we had slowly and often painfully worked out for ourselves at home, and which depended on the particular facilities there. This inevitably meant a good deal of compromise and extemporisation on holiday, which often made me wish we were back home again, among the old familiar things, and pursuing the old familiar ways.

Writing now, and looking back over some fifteen holidays spent with Mary in such circumstances, I have to confess that I can remember only the merest handful of the kind of light-hearted or comical incidents that are of the very stuff of holiday memories. I say this to my shame, for there must have been many more such occasions, the memory of which I have allowed to be blotted out by the stresses and strains of looking after Mary away from home; but there is consolation in the thought that Mary herself was probably unaware of the difficulties, and quietly got on with enjoying the change.

What of that handful of happier recollections? Undoubtedly, the happiest one of them all is of Mary, true Mum that she was, sitting talking excitedly to our daughter on the patio of her house in Germany in 1976, about the baby that Rosemary was expecting in a matter of weeks – a specially treasured image, stowed away in that 'photographic album' of my mind.

Looking back now on the mid-seventies, despite the difficulties they seem almost halcyon days. We had had that wonderful holiday in Germany in 1976, and in the early summer of 1977 we had booked a holiday in the Lake District for September of that year: it would be the furthest afield we had travelled in the car. In the meantime, apart from some constraints on her walking (she needed my arm, and managed only short distances at a time), Mary was leading a quiet but fairly normal sort of life, participating at least to some extent in most things that went on.

I remember all too well that in the middle of June 1977 she was able to attend a departmental party connected with my retirement which I was planning for later that year, taking a full part in it, and enjoying herself immensely: the photographic record of the occasion tells its own story. Indeed, as one looks at those photographs it is almost impossible to believe what awaited us, only days later, on the night of June 21st.

At that time I usually said a little prayer with Mary, after putting her to bed. Alas, in later years, and at a time when we both needed it still more, the prayer often became a casualty of our increasingly fraught circumstances. Isn't that often the case? But, perhaps, at such times, its place was taken by what the writer of *The Cloud of Unknowing* called "a naked intent" towards God – a wordless but even more urgent form of prayer.

I remember so plainly part of my prayer that night: 'The Lord make his face to shine upon you, even as you have made your face to shine upon so many.'

Four hours later Mary woke me, apparently wanting to go to the loo. It was just across the hall from what had been our dining room, but which was now our downstairs bedroom. I remember taking her the few steps across the hall and hearing her begin to say what a fine chap our younger son was. An odd thought to be expressing in the small hours, it seemed, but when she added immediately afterwards that she was so grateful, therefore, that he was now in heaven, all the horror of the realisation that she was having another stroke struck home; I had hardly got her back into bed again when she began to lose consciousness.

The doctor came, and, after examining her, he turned to me and said, "You know, if you would like me to, I could get your wife into hospital." On such occasions there are subtleties which entirely escape you, your wits blunted, and your attention gripped by the horrendous nature of what is actually going on. So I missed the point entirely and from then on we spoke at cross-purposes.

"Like this," I said, with a gesture towards Mary, "unless there is something quite specific the hospital can do for her, I want to nurse her myself, at home."

"You're quite right," he said, "and when I am in the same state, I hope someone will do the same for me."

In a daze, I asked myself a question. "Why had he said '*when* I am in the same state' and not '*if* "? But at the time, my mind, in its turmoil, could provide no answer.

That came later – as much as 24 hours later – as the full truth of Mary's condition was borne in upon me. As subtly as he could, and not realising that I had failed to understand, he had tried to tell me that Mary was dying, and that there was nothing that anybody could do for her now except to provide her with tender loving care, and save her from having to die behind the drawn curtains of a hospital bed.

My daughter-in-law Wendy arrived, almost out of thin air, like a good fairy, from Bath.

What a comfort she was, as we began the long vigil over the unconscious Mary. June 21st was a Tuesday, as my electronic calendar recently confirmed, with its solid-state accuracy; and we watched over Mary for two full days, and saw no change in her.

It got to Friday morning, and the day stretched before us with the same empty prospect of the previous two days.

Then, breaking what was literally a deathly silence, the phone bell rang. It was our doctor.

"I have been talking to the specialist at the hospital. We can't promise anything of course, but if you would agree to your wife being admitted we think there is something we can do for her, which might just work." I think he described it as 'heroic', or 'semi-heroic', whatever that meant.

He spoke cagily, almost coyly, and there was something in his manner, for whatever reason, which discouraged me from asking what it was that they were proposing to do. As a huge wave of relief broke over me, born of the previous two days of barren bleakness and inactivity, I simply said, "Of course! Of course!"

It was mid-morning, and Mary was taken straight in. At 7 o'clock in the evening Wendy and I were invited to see her.

She was sitting up in bed, seemingly more or less her old self. Typically, almost the first thing she said to me was, 'I do like your new sports jacket!' I had bought it only a few days before she was taken ill, and it had 'come out new' for her.

I was never told, and it may seem strange that I never asked, what it was they did to Mary. In particular, it has concerned me now that I hadn't asked more questions when our doctor had first rung. But that is with hindsight, and I am quite sure even after all this time that he did not encourage me – indeed that he actively discouraged me – from doing so.

I have just consulted a dictionary, and it says that 'heroic' means something 'courageous but desperate'. Was it their courage in undertaking it at all that they were being so coy about? – or was it that they thought that if they told me it would bring home to me all too plainly just how desperate Mary's situation was?

It seems that our doctor must have been very well aware that I had no illusions about Mary's plight and that it must have been to me, in fact, to whom he was offering a last glimmer of hope.

Perhaps after all, subconsciously, I realised that that was his real motive, and that was why I went along with it, asking no questions.

Perhaps too, in these matter-of-fact, materialistic days we do ask too many questions sometimes, preventing our own faith from having a chance to make its particular, and indeed unique, contribution. Mind you, such faith as I still had on that Friday morning when the doctor rang had been given to me by Mary herself, through the powers of survival she had so amply demonstrated over the years. It was a faith which, in the years that followed, was to become dangerously near to a belief that she could and would survive anything that happened to her, a belief which, however vague, carried within it the certainty of a terrible disillusionment sooner or later: it took two doctors and a nurse individually and separately, during Mary's last illness, to convince me that she was indeed dying, and that there was nothing, 'heroic', 'semi-heroic' or otherwise, that anyone could do to prevent her from doing so.

The elation we felt that Friday evening at finding Mary so suddenly and unexpectedly conscious again, and apparently her old self once more, was to be short-lived. During the ensuing days and weeks the full extent of the damage that this second stroke had caused became all too apparent. It was as though she herself experienced a brief moment of elation, only to have it brought to an abrupt end by some inner realisation that all the battles she had fought in the nine years following the first stroke had to be fought all over again; and for the time being it proved too much even for her tough spirit. Only too well do I recall another of those stark images from the 'photo album' of the mind, this time of Mary, one visiting hour, slumped like a sack of potatoes across the arm of her chair, her head actually dangling; and no-one, no-one at all, had noticed her plight. That recollection epitomises for me the month that followed the brief promise of that first Friday evening, and by the end of it I had reached a state of near-despair.

As so often happens at such times, a lifeline seemed to be thrown to me, as I stumbled on HA Williams' *True Resurrection* on my bookshelves, where it had been for two or three years without my having got around to reading it. In my spiritually near-beggared state I hungrily devoured the chapter on suffering, and restored some stamina to my failing spirit. The book, and that particular chapter, were to become a sheet anchor for me in the subsequent weeks and months of Mary's second, terrible illness.

Slowly and painfully then, I became convinced that Mary was in the wrong place – that although that particular hospital was well equipped and able to deal with an emergency such as a heart attack or a stroke, or a broken leg, it had little or nothing to offer in the way of rehabilitation, should the patient survive the initial emergency. There seemed to be no long-term plan for Mary, just extemporisation, day by day. It seemed in my overwrought state that after coping with the initial emergency, in which they had worked a near-miracle, they lost interest, or inspiration, or both. Increasingly, Mary seemed to become more and more peripheral to the mainstream of the ward's activities, out on a limb, so to say – and even something of an embarrassment; and I could stand it no longer.

I went to see a certain Dr W, who was in charge of a Rehabilitation Unit a few miles out in the country. It was housed in hutments which had been a Second World War military hospital, and first impressions of it were far from promising. But just as Mary comprised our home so, in a very real sense, did Dr W comprise that Unit – its very spirit and its life – whatever the state of dilapidation of its ageing huts.

It was, I suppose, basically a geriatric unit, something which later was to concern me greatly but briefly. Dr W had held the rank of colonel in the war, so that for him the transition from war to peace could be seen as a transition from the rehabilitation of those who had been wounded and broken down by war to rehabilitating those who had been wounded and broken down by life itself. And with what success! For in the weeks that followed it seemed to me that here indeed was a rare man, with a faith in himself and in those that worked for him that could on occasion move mountains.

The first thing that struck me about him as he fixed me with a far from idle stare across a large desk was his direct, no-nonsense manner. Discovering (I'm not sure how) that I was 'Dr' Kemp, he promptly said, "Then you are one of us." I didn't like the sound of that, fearing that it was a bit of professional snobbery, and I hastened to disabuse him, explaining that I was not a medical doctor, but that nevertheless I had spent most of my working life in the field of radiation therapy and dosimetry.

He leaned over the desk then, as though to enable him to lower his voice, and said, emphatically, almost conspiratorially, "Well, that does make you one of us, doesn't it?" I did wonder then how many medical doctors would have been prepared to concede that, and I warmed to him.

His next question, blunt, almost brusque, completely nonplussed me: "Well, now, what can I do for you?"

He must have known from Mary's notes that the stroke had scattered her to the four winds, both physically and mentally, creating massive nursing problems that made it quite out of the question for me to have her home unless and until a radical change could be brought about in her condition: and things had reached a virtual stalemate for her at the general hospital.

Despite the apparent pointlessness and insensitivity of his question, I sensed a certain subtlety underlying it, and found myself responding vigorously, and with a bluntness that matched his. "Well, you can make my wife better again just as quickly as you can, and restore her to the bosom of her family."

"Right! We know where we stand then," he responded smartly. The subtlety I had detected in his question was explained to me afterwards by our GP: I had, apparently, given him just the answer he had been looking for. So often, it seems, people went to him with the hope and intention simply of getting an aged or infirm relative taken off their hands. That, emphatically, was not how he saw his role in life: he was looking for something much more positive.

At the end of that first interview, bearing in mind that he had been the first person to show any real optimism for Mary's chances, I thanked him warmly, adding that he had done some incidental doctoring on me, too. He rounded on me again then, and with a touch of humour said, "You'd better not say things like that, or you'll get me conceited."

A retired colonel, turned medical consultant, he certainly didn't fit neatly into either of those stereotypes.

During the four months July to October 1977, I kept a private diary, spoken directly onto tape. There was no expectation at the time that the material of the diary would ever be shared with anyone other than possibly a few close members of the family, and perhaps one or two friends.

In the event it was shared with no-one at all, not even Mary, and I myself listened on one or two occasions only, to just a few fragments. In fact, it was not until August 1987 that something (I cannot remember what) prompted me to sit down and listen to all six hours of the tapes, virtually at a single session.

How then did these recordings come about in the first place? I think that it had much to do with the matter of returning home to an empty house each night, after what had often been a very difficult day, and at the end of which I had had to leave Mary behind in a hospital ward, itself overburdened with human tragedy. The recorder was, after all, something (if not *someone*) I could talk to; and so, to at least a limited extent, I could overcome the sense of aloneness created by the empty house. Of course the recorder had its drawbacks. It couldn't talk back; but, like Mary, it was a wonderful listener! – especially at the midnight hour, which as often as not it was, when I unburdened myself to it.

I talked to it, confided in it, complained to it, whispered in agony to it, cajoled it, wept and prayed in its company. In short, I dis-encumbered myself of the daily accumulation of pent-up thoughts, feelings and emotions which might otherwise have engulfed me. And there the tapes remained, and would have remained, had I not lighted upon them ten years on, and listened to them, not piecemeal but at a single sitting. It was hearing them straight through without a break that, more than anything else, changed my mind about them, and made me feel that they could and perhaps should be shared with more than a handful of family and friends.

So, during three months in the autumn of 1987, I transcribed them with as little modification as was feasible: editing out repetitive words, and occasionally repetitive thoughts; sometimes reshuffling the material recorded on a given occasion to remove incipient chaos in its ordering, and ironing out some measure of incoherence associated with the midnight hour. Thus there came into being a limited edition

– very limited! (four copies) – of a small book having the same title as the present one: one for Mary, and one for each of our three children.

During what became Mary's terminal illness, and the months that followed her death, I again resorted to tape recordings as a source of the somewhat unusual company and comfort they provided; and now, three years on, that earlier, smaller book is growing steadily into this larger one, in the attempt to give some account of the whole 20 years of Mary's quiet, heroic struggle against illness and handicap, and her as yet unsung victories over them. In this way, I hope, her victories might contribute to other victories in other places, in other lives and circumstances.

Chapter Six

It was on Thursday July 21st, exactly one month after the stroke, that Mary was transferred to the Rehabilitation Unit. Immediately prior to the move, she seemed so much more her old self again, but during her first two days in the Unit she suddenly seemed to lose a great deal of ground again, both mentally and physically. She looked so sad, and seemed bodily so much weaker. It was devastating. Many of the patients in her ward – Willow Ward – were extreme geriatric cases, and I felt sure that their plight had got through to Mary, gravely affecting her.

Rosemary was over from Germany staying with me, and we spent the whole of the Friday evening agonising over the decision I had made to allow Mary to be moved. Things seemed worse than ever for her. In the end it all became too much for us, and at ten o'clock on a Friday night I did the unthinkable, and rang up Dr W in the privacy of his own home, and gave voice to all my agony and doubt. I waited with bated breath for the inevitable burst of anger down the telephone, partly for losing faith in the Unit so quickly, but particularly for having the temerity to ring up at such an unsocial hour.

But the explosion never came, even though I plunged straight in with the thought that perhaps after all the Unit was not the right place for Mary, and that she might do better in a private nursing home somewhere, where she could have the benefit of his expertise without having to cope with what seemed to me to be the appallingly geriatric atmosphere of Willow Ward. Instead, he was the very embodiment of kindness and understanding, expressing a firm belief that the setback would prove to be a temporary one only, and predicting that Mary would quickly recover the lost ground. He spoke with quiet confidence and pride in the Unit he had built up (possibly the finest in the south of England, he said), and asked me to "give it a few more days" in which to prove itself. And when I began to apologise for ringing him up at his home, and so late at night, he interrupted me abruptly, almost impatiently, and said, "Don't apologise – as far as I am concerned, it's all part of the job."

Good-humouredly, and all sympathy, he warned me that I was "getting a bit uptight", and that I had better "start unwinding a bit". Once again I found myself comparing him with the average medic, and pondered the short shrift I might have got from such a one, in similar circumstances. What was it about the man? Was it his army training? Surely one might have expected him to pull rank in that case? No, if the army came into it at all, it was more likely for the reason that in a battle you are all in it together, facing the same odds, and with the same interest and determination to achieve a successful outcome. Rank is an irrelevance then, except as part of the overall organisation, aimed at achieving the common objective.

When I had initiated that phone call on that fateful Friday evening I had been a drowning man, engulfed in a tidal wave of horror generated by the thought of Mary caught up in the unrelieved and seemingly unrelievable tragedies of Willow Ward. It says a great deal for Dr W's powers of persuasion and his own faith in his hand-picked team that as I put the phone down that wave of horror had been very largely dissipated. I had a lot more to learn about Willow Ward than I knew, that Friday evening.

In the event, it was the ward staff who saw to it that I met the geriatric aspects of Willow Ward head-on. It was not that they adopted any special tactics on my behalf – they simply went about their business, behaving as they had always done, not aware of my problems. Why should they be? – as far as one could tell they themselves had none at all, not of the kind I had, anyway. From the start it was obvious that they deeply enjoyed their work. A vein of real humour was never far below the surface, and despite the sombre circumstances there was often real fun in the air. And it was that, more than anything else, that brought about my Damascus Road experience regarding the care of the frankly senile. It cannot be doubted that behind all that was done by the staff in Willow Ward there was a great deal of expertise, perhaps of their own, or of Dr W's special brand. Even so, I am sure that it was the spirit in which their work was carried out which counted most towards their spectacular successes, which had earned the Unit its reputation and which, in Mary's case, ultimately amounted to little short of a miracle.

Generalities are useless to describe what I mean: some actual incidents will speak for themselves.

There was the occasion when young Gary, who was one of the kitchen staff, was asked to take one of the old ladies a cup of tea, but finding her on the bed with her head hanging down and her legs in the air he commented archly that he wasn't sure that it was right for her to have a cup of tea in that position. Without a sign of the bustling, no-nonsense efficiency of a general hospital ward, which, in the case of old people, can certainly have its drawbacks, he quietly dealt with her, and duly gave her her cup of tea.

It was Gary, too, who, receiving a complaint about the smell of the prunes that were cooking in the kitchen, emerged with an air freshener spray, and proceeded to fill the ward with the scent of it, only to have the neglected prunes burn dry, and their smell, far worse than the original smell of the cooking prunes, took over the whole place – something which he was certainly not allowed to forget in a hurry.

Then there was the old lady who was under the illusion that she was staying in a hotel, and who one day continually addressed one nurse as "waitress". In the end the nurse stomped down the ward in mock indignation, saying that she had been called all sorts of things in her job, but never "waitress" before.

There was the day, too, when I found ants on Mary's bedside locker, and gingerly mentioned them to Gary (the ward was, after all, housed in a prefab hut, and the weather was hot, and the windows and doors wide open). He took one look at them, and instead of some official (not to say officious) reaction, he straightened himself and said, "Really, you've been let off quite lightly, you know. You should see them in the rest of the ward." And as if to point the issue he added, "And you should see the ones in the Nurses' Home – they're gigantic ones, from outer space in fact." With no more ado then, he went off to get the ant powder. Even this was described to me in mock sci-fi terms by the nurses, who insisted that it was the very latest thing, which caused the ants to eat each other. And all this was going on in the middle of what would otherwise have been a tense meal-time situation, with its special problems in a geriatric ward.

Later still, one of the nurses was trying to mop up some stewed tomatoes with one of those standard government-issue mops with its foot-long tassels, and was being thoroughly scathing about its uselessness for such a purpose. She ended up with a box of paper tissues, much more effective in clearing up the mess. All this went on with many a jocular aside to the old lady responsible for the spillage in the first place, the nurse saying at one point that she was going to teach her to use the mop for herself, so that she could clear up her own tomatoes in future.

If all this gaiety of spirit and lightness of touch had not been so obviously spontaneous, I would have been tempted to believe that it originated in some edict or other stemming from Dr W himself. I think not, though I have no doubt that it ultimately stemmed from him – from the way in which he hand-picked his staff, from the highly qualified nurses right down to those who worked in the kitchens. Come to think of it, why should I say 'right down to'? As we have already seen, Dr W never stood on his dignity and was no respecter of persons; he would have chosen his staff to form a homogeneous team of like-minded people having the same spirit and lightness of touch across the whole gamut of activities making up the daily round of the ward. That I believe, even 14 years on, to have been the main plank of his success.

It was certainly at the root of the subtle alchemy Willow Ward worked on me during those first few, vital days of Mary's stay there. To begin with, to my tired spirit, such apparent levity seemed totally out of place, but I quickly came to realise that the fun and laughter of those young people was an important part of the caring and indeed the *healing* art which they practised round the clock, transforming the atmosphere in which those old, and in some cases desperately senile patients were living out their last days; totally transforming, too, that appalling impact which Willow Ward had had on me initially. So much so that they soon had me laughing with them, as they went about their tasks. And that did me a power of good, too.

It has been said that laughter is the quintessentially human quality. HA Williams, in his little volume called *Tensions*, has argued that laughter "is the best and clearest reflection we ever get in this world of God's love for his creation," adding that "in laughter we see the Celestial City in what is more than a passing glimpse." Is Harry Williams implying that laughter is of the very nature of God? What a thought!

Willow Ward started to get through to Mary, too, just as Dr W had predicted, and she began to stir again, both physically and mentally. Thus, on the Sunday following that vital phone call, she quite suddenly found herself able to lift both feet right up, to enable me to move the bedside table close to her – and this just a week after my being told at the general hospital that "her legs just don't belong to her."

"Just look at that!" I said.

"Yes, isn't it wonderful?" she replied, quietly.

It was on that Sunday, too, that I rang up after breakfast, and was told a little coyly by the ward sister that I could go over at lunchtime if I wanted to, but if I had it in mind that it would be to help, that would not be necessary as, at breakfast, Mary had fed herself – the first time that she had fed herself since being taken ill.

It might be argued that these things would have happened anyway, Willow Ward or no Willow Ward. I don't believe that. Sometimes, just sometimes, we are aware that common events have taken an uncommon turn, and that common things have taken on a distinctly uncommon aura. Yet, after all these years, I still find it difficult to fit a word to that secret ingredient that was part of all that went on in Willow Ward. Do I really, though, find it so difficult? Isn't the problem simply that there is indeed a word that fits precisely, but that it is one whose currency has been grossly devalued these days, to the point where we hesitate to use it, lest it clouds rather than clarifies?

Love has a currency
All its own:
Its smallest denomination
Is of inestimable worth –
Yet it is theft-proof,
And thus needs no protection.

Minted freely,
It creates no fear of inflation –
In fact, it reverses
All the usual rules.

Thus, unless it is counterfeit,
Its investment
Seeks no return;
And income actually increases
With expenditure.

Its nature is always to be
A gift –
It cannot therefore be earned,
Or claimed as any kind of recompense
Or reward;
And, when returned,
It needs to be immediately reinvested;
For the attempt to hoard it
Leads to bankruptcy.

It defies
Drawing up a balance sheet,
For it cannot be enumerated;
And any attempt
To put a price on it
Renders it worthless.
It is always available on demand,
And requires no security:
Indeed,
It may take the form
Of a blank cheque,
With the consequences
Willingly accepted;
For counting the cost
Is foreign to it.

It is exchangeable
The world over,
But such exchange
Must always be
Person to person:
No broker
Can have dealings in it
To achieve a cheap gain.

It can be taxed
To the limit,
Yet emerge
With enhanced reserves:
It is the only currency
Adequate to meet the cost
Of living.

I have no doubt myself that the fun and the laughter and the lightness of touch which characterised the whole life of Willow Ward was the very catalyst enabling love to work its seeming miracles without overwhelming the giver or the receiver. Perhaps that is why God himself needs laughter – to veil the intensity of his love?

TS Eliot has said that Man can stand only a little reality at one time, and perhaps that is even true of the quintessence of life, which we call love.

Many years ago a friend said to me, "You know, life gives you a pat on the back one day, and a smack on the bottom the next."

Hardly appropriate words for Willow Ward days, but in substance a fair comment on the weeks and months that were to follow that first brief, heady time, when so much seemed to be coming together for Mary. But I was going to have to learn the hard way that despite the initial steep gains that followed the setbacks of the first two days, progress in general was going to be very much an up-and-down affair, a process inherent in the very nature of Mary's problems.

How well I remember Thursday, July 28th, exactly one week after her admission to the Unit, and the day that had preceded it. I was on Cloud Nine that Wednesday. Mary showed little or no trace of confusion all day, and fed herself completely: she also seemed to have very good movement in her legs. I had been out to the shops and bought her a very pretty button-through summer dress, which she was wearing when I got there. In fact, the visiting hairdresser had just given her a shampoo and wave when I arrived and, not to put too fine a point on it, she looked absolutely smashing. As I wheeled her back down the ward between the two rows of beds I deliberately cracked a joke (her ability to recognise humour and to respond to it had been one of the subtler victims of the stroke). I said to her that she looked positively regal, and ought to be giving the royal salute. To my delight she actually giggled, for the first time since the stroke – and what music *that* was to my ears.

There were other 'first times', too, that I noticed that Wednesday. It was the day on which Mary once more seemed to be able to make a meaningful choice between two alternatives. We don't give a second thought to that sort of thing when things are normal, but the fact is that up till then, faced with even the simplest of choices, Mary had looked pathetically blank, as though making a choice (and indeed the nature of choice itself) was beyond her very ken. Thus, I noticed that she immediately chose between two dessert courses offered to her at supper-time. And again, when I was putting away her handbag in one part of her locker she suddenly said, "No, don't put it there, put it lower down." A little thing, trivial, to the point of insignificance, not worth mentioning? Oh, yes! – well worth it, when one has been clutching frantically at every straw in a field harvested of almost every grain of comfort, as I had been doing, for a whole month.

Mary looked so sweet as I left her that Wednesday night, and I was looking forward so much to 'showing her off' to her brother, who was taking the opportunity of a business visit from the North to London to come out to see her. He had been in a fortnight earlier, when she had been such a forlorn and pathetic sight at the general hospital, and I was sure he would see such a difference in her.

Alas, the realities of that Thursday fell so far short of my expectations for it. All Mary's clarity of thought and speech had forsaken her. She was what the medics would have described as thoroughly confused again, and strangely euphoric too, as she had been, to some extent, from time to time ever since the stroke. It was a bizarre combination which horrified me, even though she looked quite well and fed herself throughout her supper.

I was somewhat comforted, as I left the hospital with her brother, to hear him say how much better he had found her compared with his previous visit; and I realised that my perspective was bound to be distorted by my very closeness to Mary, and as a result of seeing her two or three times a day as I was doing. Even so, last thing that night, and alone again, I was heavy of heart, and took myself out for a walk in the dark in which, in some strange way, I found comfort and solace.

HA Williams, in *True Resurrection*, says, "Suffering always involves aloneness, a being cut off from others" – an experience which daytime, with all the busy life of the world going on about us, seems to emphasise. Harry Williams goes on: "While all our human resources are being press-ganged by the dead weight of suffering, other people are laughing, drinking in the pub, making love, or planning tomorrow's picnic." Or, as I myself had put it in some lines written years before, after Mary's first stroke:

> The world goes by:
> Young lovers kiss
> In the streets;
> And ageing couples
> Saunter,
> Scanning the windows
> For bargains
> In tomorrow's sales;
> Old people sit,
> Slightly apart,
> On the seats;
> And young bloods
> Thunder past
> Astride their machines,
> Thirsting for trouble,
> Oblivious, all,
> Of the miracle
> Of arms
> And legs,
> And simple conversation.

With the coming of night, the day's activity dies down; and one is much less aware of the life that is all about us and thus of feeling excluded from it.

Darkness seemed to be a positive balm to my spirit that evening, inducing a contemplative mood; and as I walked I found all my complex wishes and desires being reduced to the simplest of all – that Mary and I might be 'restored' to each other, whatever that might come to mean for us in the days that lay ahead.

And there I left it as I turned homeward, with the hardest thing of all still to be faced – that of coming to terms for yet another night with having had to leave Mary in a hospital ward several miles away, in the charge of others.

The next morning the whole cosmic problem of suffering was with me still, and one of Richard Harries' *Prayers of Hope* ('God Doesn't Will Suffering') came to mind. He deals first with the argument that God does sometimes will suffering upon us in order to bring out qualities such as courage or patience, thus fitting us the more fully for the eternal harmony and bliss of some 'hereafter'. Like Harry Williams, Richard Harries quotes Ivan in *The Brothers Karamozov* who, confronted with the indescribable cruelty to a young child inflicted on it by its cultured parents, protests that the attainment of any such harmony and bliss "is not worth the tears of one tortured child [who] prays with its unexpatiated tears to 'dear kind God' ... I protest, "(says Ivan) "that the truth is not worth such a price."

"What then can a Christian say?" asks Harries. "There is no conclusive human answer to the question why in a world made by a good God there is so much evil and suffering, and some answers are quite out of the question, but" (and this is the point, says Harries) "when we are at the end of our tether, when we feel oppressed and got down by life, when all human resources fail, there is still what Paul called 'a power that worketh within us' ... What the disciples experienced after the crucifixion can be experienced now, and most particularly at those times when we feel most completely defeated."

Of that "power" I have no earthshaking, headline-grabbing examples to report, but I am convinced that at crucial moments in my own life, when "all human resources have failed", and I have felt "most completely defeated", help has been forthcoming, not in any spectacular mode or manner, but simply as guidance which has proved crucial, coming almost incidentally, often via a few words, spoken seemingly casually, or leaping out from a printed page which I had stumbled on in a desperate search for help.

Thus was it during Mary's month in the general hospital, when, in the deep dusk of a summer's evening, and the deep dark of near-desperation, I had come upon Harry Williams' *True Resurrection*, neglected, on my own bookshelves; and, in an exactly similar fashion and state of mind, after Mary's death, I took from my shelves Martin Israel's *The Pain That Heals*, bought several years before, and unread till then.

That breakfast-time in 1977 was typical of many during the 20 years of Mary's illnesses when, at the beginning of a new day, some aspect of her handicaps would strike me afresh as so unfair and undeserved, viewed from any ordinary standpoint based on ethics, morality, justice, logic, or whatever other system of thought or reasoning happened to present itself over a plate of cornflakes. As Harry Williams argues, there is no answer to the problem of suffering along any such lines. "We could say that explaining facts is an attempt to soften their impact upon us. For the explanation is felt as a sort of exorcism which casts out some at least of the sheer brutality of the fact. It is thus that we escape from life into theory, from experience into doctrine, from the thing itself into talk about it."

It was to be another ten years before I stumbled on what was for me to be the most simple and profoundly satisfying resolution of this whole matter, embodied in a little homily on Radio 4 at Christmastide in 1987, just months before Mary died.

Chapter Seven

As I got to know Willow Ward better I came to realise that underneath the apparent lightheartedness, seemingly carried to the point almost of haphazardness at times, there lay a hardheaded realism that brooked no shallow optimism whatsoever. Time and again, clutching at a straw, I would wax enthusiastic about some little improvement I had detected in Mary, only to have my undue hopefulness immediately tempered by a firm note of caution deliberately calculated to bring me back to earth, and with something of a bump too, if deemed necessary.

An early example of this was on Sunday July 31st, three days after Mary's brother's visit when she had, it seemed, quickly picked up again. The day before, she had staggered me by offering to walk a little, as I was preparing to get her wheel chair ready. I was convinced that she was a little confused again, and hotfooted it to Sister, who said coyly, "Oh, yes, she can walk a little – that is, with some support on either side."

It was a little surprise that they had cooked up for me between the two of them; so that, on the Sunday, when I went over at lunchtime with Rosemary, we were quite prepared to believe them when they told us that she had walked the whole length of the ward that morning.

Mentally, she seemed so improved too – able to read several pages of a book at a sitting, and holding her own in a series of questions and answers, with no signs of confusion. I well remember wondering excitedly what Dr W would think of her on his ward round the next day, if she was as well as that still and he was told, additionally, that she was walking again.

I had dropped to a part-time working routine by then, but Monday was one of my working days, so I would have to wait until the evening to find out how things had gone. When I got over to the Unit for Mary's supper-time she was just a tiny bit confused, and showing some compulsive behaviour (which always distressed me), but otherwise she seemed quite nicely. However, when I asked her whether Dr W had seen her she first of all said "Yes" and then subsequently "No" so that in the end I had to ask Sister as I left.

She said, rather noncommittally, "Yes, he has been."

I sensed her reticence, and asked her with some trepidation whether he had said anything.

She, in her turn, sensed that I was hanging on her every word, and looked a little downhearted then. "Well, your wife was quite confused today when he saw her, and she didn't want to walk, either." Then she added, almost as an afterthought it seemed, that it was perhaps because there had been only one person there to help.

Desperately I clutched at a straw again, though my spirits were plummeting. "That might well have been the reason," I responded. "Ever since her first stroke she has had a quite understandable, though untoward, fear of falling."

Sister nodded in agreement, but went on to say that when Mary was confused it made it more difficult for her to take instructions, and that was bound to slow things up. Weighing up my mood then, she cautioned me that it was "going to be a long time." Even as she spoke, I knew that it was a coded message – that she was telling me that if Mary's confusion didn't finally clear up, she might never be able to cooperate enough to respond adequately to the rehabilitation programme.

That night, home again and alone, I was back with my old heartache, back with the need to keep at arm's length the purely medical prognoses, back with the need to regenerate the hope and faith that had permeated the weekend in spite of Sister's pessimism; and back with the sheer necessity of being prepared to swim against the stream, for Mary's sake.

The next day was August 2nd, our wedding anniversary. I sent her what I hoped she would feel was a happy little note, wrested from the desolation that had all too easily taken possession of me again that night.

A party of students from the general hospital where Mary had spent that first month was being shown round the Rehabilitation Unit. I had gone over for Mary's lunchtime, and was approaching Willow Ward when a young West Indian nurse broke away from the rest of the party and came rushing up to me. She threw her arms round me, and I thought for a moment that she was actually going to kiss me.

She was all smiles, and bubbling with enthusiasm. "Hasn't your wife got on wonderfully!" she exclaimed.

And what had thrilled her more than anything was that when Mary had first spotted her as they were being shown round Willow Ward she had shouted out joyfully, "Oh, look! There's my nurse!"

She had been on Mary's ward, and Mary had grown very attached to her during that otherwise barren month; and there is little doubt that losing her had contributed to Mary's early setback at the Unit.

Mary's greeting says it all, and was so typical of the way in which she related to all those who served her needs, and cared for her in whatever way: nurses, doctors, physiotherapists, occupational therapists, ward maids, nursing auxiliaries – there was nearly always one whom she would adopt from each group and thereafter refer to as hers, upon whom she would bestow her affection so generously, and so subtly.

There were others, many others. There was another West Indian nurse, for instance, who was on Willow Ward and who, one evening when I was sitting with Mary, came over to us, just after putting a tape on in the ward. It was what would be called 'country style' I think, and she said shyly that she had dedicated it to us. I am sure she meant Mary really. I couldn't tell what the words were, so I went over and inspected the tape itself, to find that the title was 'I Won't Forget You Now'.

And it was she who, on a previous evening, had peered between the curtains to see how we were getting on, only to discover me giving Mary a kiss, and had said discreetly, "Sorry! I'll come back later"!

There was the young Mauritian male nurse too, who was adopted by Mary in her usual fashion, and in his turn adopted me: in some special sort of way, I seemed to become *in loco parentis* to him. I say "Mauritian", as I had been told that he "came from Mauritius", and assumed that he was a native thereof. Ingenuously enough, then, but with a typically humorous touch, he made me aware of my mistake.

They were playing a tape of some traditional Indian music, and I asked him if he liked the music. Looking at the other nurses then, he said, with a glint in his eye, "Don't throw stones at me." He was from South India.

Whenever I appeared on the ward, if there was the opportunity he would join me at Mary's bedside, and chatter eagerly about all manner of things. He found out that it was only late in life that I had learned to drive, and that, despite that, I had taken the Advanced Driving Test. He cross-examined me then as to why I had bothered to do so, and for that sole reason came to regard me as some sort of oracle on motorcars and motoring, to my great embarrassment. He would quiz me endlessly (he was shortly to take his test) until finally he was ticked off in a good-natured manner by Staff Nurse for not getting on with his work. But in truth they were all past masters at balancing the serious business of the ward against the occasional bit of light relief. I am convinced that it was uniquely helpful to both the staff and the patients, and it was surely one of the secrets of their success.

Typical of the informality which characterised the work of the ward was the occasion when the young Mauritian, passing the end of Mary's bed, gave her the 'Thumbs Up' sign, at the same time raising his eyebrows in a query, as much as to say, 'Everything OK?', and to his delight and mine she replied with a simple 'Thumbs up' of her own. At a time when Mary was still having great difficulties communicating in whatever manner, how I cherished that little incident as evidence of her further progress!

One final delightful touch of Mary's, triggered by a little bit of banter by the young Mauritian: in front of Mary he said to me, "You know, Sister has got rather a soft spot for you," and I said, "Well, as a matter of fact, I've got rather a soft spot for Sister." And Mary, quick as a flash, butted in, archly, "I think it is time we were going home then!"

But perhaps the most important of all those whom Mary adopted was 'my physiotherapist' – Miss R, the one who, probably more than anyone else on the Unit, was instrumental in "restoring Mary to the bosom of her family", as I had put it to Dr W, in that memorable first interview with him.

My first interview with Miss R proved memorable for another reason – we discovered that I had taught her physics at The London Hospital some 20 years before. What a small world it turns out to be sometimes; and what a tangled web of relationships is sometimes woven by fortuitous events.

Tangled and fortuitous though the events might have been that had brought us together again, I felt there was a special bond between us that augured well for the future. When I had known her at The London Hospital she had been just one of a sea of faces in a lecture room, but at the Rehabilitation Unit it was quite another matter. On two separate occasions I remember describing her as a "steaming cauldron of enthusiasm"; and again, as a "veritable fireball". Her enthusiasm on Mary's behalf was such that she swept me along with it, and I was soon serving an accelerated apprenticeship with her in regard to all sorts of manipulations and practical procedures which were to stand us in good stead when Mary was home again. Not everyone, though, was as enthusiastic as I was about Miss R's drive and energy. As one patient put it to me, "If you've been in the army you know what it is to have to deal with the sergeant major." But he said it with a twinkle in his eye.

Miss R spared Mary nothing, and for that matter spared me nothing either. Some of the things that went on seemed positively brutal. For instance, she would get Mary to lie on her back, and then to turn her head to one side or the other. It was for me, then, to roll first her shoulders and then her hips over, in the direction in which she was looking. Mary was absolutely terrified of this exercise, but Miss R said that it was these things (of which Mary was afraid) that were particularly good for her: fear was indicative of a sense of insecurity which had gradually got to be overcome by getting her to do these things until she was confident, and so lost her fears. This particular theory of Miss R's was wonderfully illustrated and substantiated on Mary's very first night home – but that story needs to be told in its proper context.

Another example: Mary hated leaning forward, so Miss R got her to clasp her hands together, lean on her elbows on a table, and then push her arms across it as far as she could go. Soon I was being asked to remove the table, and before we knew where we were Mary, hands still clasped, was standing up and walking a few steps without her frame. And how subtle so much of this was! Apparently, clasping her hands together in that way as she walked helped to prevent her right leg from going into spasm – which in turn helped to prevent her from raising her right foot off the floor when she first stood. Otherwise she might have ended up almost hopping along!

The only encouragement Mary needed through all this was the knowledge that everything she mastered for Miss R got her a step nearer to going home.

Attention to every conceivable detail was another of Miss R's specialities. For example, I assured her that we had a commode of our own, and would not need a "Health Service issue", but she insisted on my taking it in one day for her scrutiny, and when she saw it, she promptly offered to pad the seat for us. There is more to that story later, too!

I well remember coming across her one morning, just as she arrived. She clambered out of her car with a characteristic gleam in her eye and said that while she had been driving in she had been thinking about the problems we would face when Mary was home again, and had recalled a device which she thought would be the very thing for us: she was confident that it would solve most of the problems of getting Mary to stand, and to be able to continue standing, while I attended to her – for example to dress and undress her. The device, called a 'Stand Easy', apparently looked something like a child's scooter (with fixed handlebars and no wheels), and though probably unavailable under the Health Service could be purchased direct from the manufacturers. One got the continual impression that once Miss R was awake (though by no means necessarily up and dressed), her mind was already on her patients and their problems, and remained there until she was actually in bed again at night.

Finally, jumping well ahead in the story, there was Miss R's visit home, immediately prior to Mary's return. She had brought a wheelchair, which was to be on loan to us, and had taken the opportunity to look round the house to inspect the preparations I had made for Mary's homecoming, from the removal of all rugs and the laying of carpet tiles wherever necessary, to the installation of a washing machine and spin drier. She ended up in the kitchen, looking a little pensive for her, usually so ebullient. Suddenly she said, "Of course, what all our patients need is the love and the care of one person. Sometimes they can have the love, and sometimes the care: the problem is to have them both in the same person."

The remark was a far cry from mere physiotherapy.

It should not be concluded from all this that Mary received any kind of preferential treatment whilst she was in Willow Ward. From my own observations over those weeks, all the patients (including those whose state of extreme senility had almost overwhelmed me in the early days) were equal beneficiaries from the tender loving care lavished without limit upon them by the staff. And it was through my close involvement in the life of the ward, often three times a day, that I was made to realise the lovable qualities of many of even the worst cases (I've done it myself now: it makes life so much simpler if you think of 'cases' rather than 'people'). Take the 'case' of the old lady opposite Mary, who was so obstreperous at times. After only a few days of participating in the life of the ward I was talking to her, stroking her hair. She was so nice, and blew me a kiss as I left her.

Then there was the little old Scottish lady, who had been so thrilled with Rosemary's one-year-old when we took him over for Mary to see. I told her he was beginning to say "Mamma" and "Daddy", and she said, "Ee! they do bring them on young these days." Alas, it was not often that the inmates of Willow Ward got the chance to come under the spell of a one-year-old (and how therapeutic it must have been!)

But the plight of the old lady in the next bed to Mary's was a sad comparison. One day she told me of a family quarrel that had gone on at her bedside the night before. There had been an attempt to sell off some land against her wishes. Poor old soul – somehow she had sensed my academic background and added bitterly, "You professors [sic] – you should do something about the indignity of old age."

Chapter Eight

It would be quite inappropriate to say of Mary's recovery that it came together, brick by brick, like a building taking shape, each brick recognizable for what it was, and taking its place neatly with all the others, in accordance with the architect's plans. Quite the contrary: flexibility, a readiness to change direction and to extemporise, were surely all part of the master plan behind the running of Willow Ward. This included a willingness to recognise that having looked after Mary for so long, and being able to spend so much more time with her than the staff could possibly do, I was in a position to become aware of the subtler changes that were taking place in her which might have escaped the staff.

There were the much more subtle, personal things, too, so vital to me, representing as they did a returning sense in Mary of 'belonging' to us all again.

One evening, after she had been in the Unit about a fortnight, during most of which time she had been (as I used to put it) "scattered to the four winds", she suddenly said, just as I was leaving, "We've been kind of cut off, haven't we?"

I said, "Yes, love, but we're not so any longer, are we?"

And with huge enthusiasm she replied, "Oh, no!"

What a 'goodnight kiss' that was!

Again, one afternoon, as I said "Goodbye", adding that I would be back in the evening, out of the blue she said, quietly and seriously, "And how are you?"

"I'm OK," I responded, as casually as maybe, sensing real concern behind the question.

She looked hard at me then and smiled, and to my amazement said, "You've got what it takes, haven't you?"

"So have you!" I fired back, "and that makes two of us!"

It wasn't the sentiment itself that struck me, but her newly acquired ability to express it so subtly, after struggling for a single word sometimes, in which to express anything at all.

Such moments of lucidity were not always happy ones, however – far from it. There was the evening when she greeted me so gently as I arrived, saying that she had a question for me. I took it light-heartedly, as some sort of joke she had dreamed up on my behalf, and said, "Fire away, then!" But she asked me, so terribly wistfully, how soon I thought it would be before she was able to think about her "waterworks" again, as she put it.

It all but broke my heart – she looked so sad as she asked the question. I hastened to tell her not to worry. What else could I have said? – I didn't want her to start having worries about it, on top of the problem itself.

As if to underline it all, just before I left that night they discovered her nightie was wet. She hadn't any more of her own, so they got a sort of outsize pyjama top from the ward cupboard and put it on her, and she looked such a poor waif in it: it was awful having to leave her, looking like that. Yet, in the midst of all this turmoil, one had to be thankful that she was beginning to be able to express herself again, her thoughts, her feelings, and her worries – to ask questions about them, and to have enough concentration again, to be able to consider the answers.

I still have a close-lined four-page letter written by Mary in 1974 to an aged aunt of hers. For some reason or other it never got sent. It is beautifully written, with her left hand, well constructed, wonderfully anecdotal, and almost beyond credulity now. Why? – because, immediately after the 1977 stroke she could not put a single meaningful sentence together on paper, even though her speech, by comparison, was only slightly affected. It was for this reason that, during those early weeks in the Rehabilitation Unit, I looked eagerly for any signs of improvement in this area.

There came the time when one evening I noticed her ball pen on the table, and I said diffidently, "Have you been trying out your writing?"

She grimaced a little. "Well – I haven't made much of a go of it."

Not to be put off, I produced the proverbial back of an envelope, and asked her to try again. She started to write what looked like a shopping list, albeit a somewhat quaint one, "Three ounces of marmalade, one Danish loaf...", written with her left hand, almost as fast as any writing she had done since that first stroke, in 1968. How marvellous I thought it was, that she should again be able to perform such a complex operation as writing, within two months of having the second stroke. But it was to prove a disappointment, for although, a few days later, she wrote a little, single-sentence letter to Rosemary in Germany (so memorable at the time that I photographed it), followed a little later by a two-sentence letter to our son John in Canterbury, it was progress that was not to be maintained.

Thus, years later, her writing ability was still capricious, totally unpredictable. Sometimes she would manage to put a few sentences together, which were both comprehensible and reasonably fluent, but at other times, though she herself would seem satisfied with what she had written, it was little more than gobbledygook. There were times, indeed, when I had to go through the motions of posting a letter whilst refraining from actually doing so, so distressing might it have been to the recipient.

In the end, the time came when I dreaded to hear Mary say that she was going to write a letter.

However, it was a very different matter with her reading. As with almost everything else, her ability to concentrate on the printed word had been gravely diminished. So much so that the first books I took her when she had been transferred to the Unit were to all intents and purposes 'picture books', the one a book of beautiful landscape photographs, illustrating quotations from the Psalms, and the other a book of cartoons by Thelwell, called *Down the Garden Path*. The idea was that in their respective ways the pictures in both these books would generate enough interest in themselves to encourage Mary to become interested again in the words that accompanied them. And so it turned out, though to begin with it was I who had to read them to her!

Only ten days later, she was reading several pages of a book at a sitting, and a week later still I came upon her hidden behind *The Guardian*, absorbed in an inner page. The following Sunday, after Mary's roast beef, roast potatoes, and Yorkshire pudding, found us like old times, each with our own bit of *The Observer*, just as we used to be at home. And all this within a month of her being admitted to the Unit.

Only ten days further on, and I bought her a copy of *The Ragged-trousered Philanthropists*, confident that she was ready to tackle a really long book once more.

Mary's ability to concentrate again, and her restored interest in reading, were to prove vital to her for it was reading, above all else, that was to fill her remaining days.

Any account of Mary's progress towards that moment which bisected time for us, when it was agreed that at least on a trial basis she could come home again must, inevitably, be largely anecdotal.

The daily routines of the ward were methodical, but for the rest, to be sure, there was much that was truly inspirational. It is significant how often it has been necessary to use words that would look more at home in a religious context than a medical one – 'love', 'spirit', 'miracle', 'faith', and the like – but to have tried to avoid them would have been to distort the truth about Willow Ward and the man who there waged his continuing battle against the march of time in the lives of those in his charge.

Where to start then, among all the seemingly kaleidoscopic events that led up to Mary's homecoming? Perhaps not with any particular event at all, but rather with the realisation that the whole sequence occupied 5 weeks only – just 35 days.

"The impossible takes a little longer," it used to be said, and it took Dr W and his team just 4 days longer than the month Mary had spent languishing in the general hospital, to transform her from a pathetic bundle of total misery and almost-total inertia to someone so very much nearer her old self again. She could think plainly, talk plainly, feed herself, read well, and walk again. It is true that she had many problems still. She could still get confused, still fail to find the right word, was still incontinent, and still needed a caliper and a walking frame. But they were all problems that could be coped with, given a bit of forethought and organisation.

And it was not only Mary that had been transformed. I had undergone a sea change too. under the spell of Willow Ward. I also had been a bundle if not of misery then of near-hopelessness and worse.

Recalling again that memory of Mary slumped over the arm of a chair, her head and the whole of the top half of her body dangling helplessly, with no-one even to notice her plight, I know now that I must have had grave doubts about the wisdom of that "semi-heroic" action I had agreed to so enthusiastically a month before. Indeed, it had already come under some question when I had told our GP how euphoric Mary tended to be: his reply had been that he was only too grateful that "it hadn't gone the other way", as he put it – that she wasn't weeping all day long.

Had it really been as haphazard, as chancey as all that – a terrible, awesome gamble on Mary's behalf, with her having no choice at all in the matter, the whole thing resting on a simple "Aye" or "Nay" from me? The responsibility I took upon myself that Friday morning when I agreed to her going into hospital (so naively, it seems now) seems almost unbearable in retrospect. In mitigation, it must be reiterated that the considerations were never spelled out to me and, at the time, it never even occurred to me to ask.

And, in truth, the Mary that came home from Willow Ward was, *by comparison*, so much more able to enjoy her life again, so much more within my capabilities to look after, her life so much more sustainable, that it was hardly likely to occur to me to question the decision afterwards.

"By comparison," – comparison, that is, with the Mary who, in the general hospital, was drooping steadily and withering away before my eyes, like a plant that badly needed watering. But by comparison with the Mary that took three A levels with good credits at the age of 58? That is a question I have only just begun to dare to ask.

It was Monday, August 8th, and Mary had been in the Unit two and a half weeks – just half her total stay, as it turned out to be. And over that weekend I had been taking stock.

It was on the preceding Friday that Mary had said "We've been kind of cut off, haven't we?" – that remarkably subtle assessment of how things had been for us, bearing in mind that only a week or so before she had hardly been able to string even two or three words together to make any kind of sense.

There were other things, too. It was that Friday evening when I had plucked up courage to ask about breakfast-times. I had become all too aware of the paucity of her short-term memory, and had learned to avoid the unnecessary and sometimes bitter disappointments which resulted from testing out her weak spots, in the hope of gleaning some fresh crumb of comfort or encouragement. But genuine curiosity about how the day began for her (I was never there at breakfast-time!) and some subconscious hunch that it was a good moment to ask, gave me the confidence to pop the question – did they give her breakfast in bed, or did they get her up first?

It was the kind of question, offering a choice of answers, that only days before she would have found impossible to understand, let alone answer.

"Oh, no!" she exclaimed, without any hesitation. "They get us up in our chairs first, and then they bring us breakfast."

Then again, as the supper trolley emerged from the kitchen, and enormously encouraged by her response, I said, "It smells like fish again – surely it can't be!"

Her reply was as prompt and as positive as the previous one. "No – it can't be, because I had grilled haddock for lunch."

Alas, one who, reading these words, is

Oblivious, all,
Of the miracle
Of simple conversation,

will not be able to appreciate the sheer joy of this little exchange. Little wonder that Mary herself had said, as I left that evening, "We've been kind of cut off, haven't we?"

But there had been other things too: her ability to feed herself, particularly coming to use a fork properly again (she had lost all idea of 'spearing' food with it); her first attempts at writing; and beginning to walk again, albeit with the aid of a caliper and walking frame; above all else her ability to relate to me for a couple of hours on end, almost as though she had never had a second stroke.

It was enough. And on that Monday morning, and just as I had done on the Friday evening a fortnight before, I plucked up courage and rang Dr W at his home again, just after breakfast. I spelled out my assessment of Mary's progress as I saw it and of her ability to be more or less her old self again for an hour or two on end.

There is no doubt that he felt his role to be one of damping down what he saw as my over-ardent expectations of Mary, and his reply was characteristic.

"Well, wait another three weeks, then ring again, and I'll give you another assessment."

It certainly worked, and it was in a suitably subdued frame of mind that I entered the ward, three hours later.

Sister had been lying in wait for me, and to my astonishment she told me that on the strength of my phone call Dr W had made a beeline for Mary, and, instead of another assessment in three weeks, he was talking now of a possible homecoming in that time – or even earlier, if they could find an answer to the incontinence problem; and she commissioned me there and then to work on it with Mary.

How thrilled she was! – her whole face radiant on our behalf at the mere thought that some sort of time-scale had at last been put on Mary's homecoming. Had she really begun to think that it was never to be?

The next day I took a day's leave from work, and went over early to the Unit, feeling that there might be some sort of action filtering down from Dr W's reassessment. There was. First Miss R, and then the occupational therapist, asked to see me in turn to discuss matters generally, and to demonstrate certain things in particular, all directed to Mary's homecoming. There was no fuss. It was like a change of gear in an automatic car – that it had taken place was evident from the change of speed, and the sounds coming from the engine, but the actual gear change had been almost imperceptible. Neither was any significant time spent or energy expended on discussing Mary's new prospects: it was a case of eyes straight ahead through the windscreen, with no time to look at the change of scenery through the side windows. To change the metaphor altogether, it was as though an Alert had been sounded, not to an imminent threat of danger, but to the unexpected promise of victory. The galvanizing effect on the staff had been just the same, however.

From that time on everything changed, and became subtly geared to Mary's homecoming. And this was true, not only of what went on in the Unit on Mary's behalf – I found my own modest contribution changing too. I asked if I could take Mary round the grounds in a wheel chair when the weather was suitable, and this became a daily routine. It enabled her to break out from the microcosm of the ward, and to appreciate again that there was a world outside and beyond, which included home and family. It was at this time that I wheeled her to the car, opened the passenger door, waved my hand towards the seat, and announced that that was where she would soon be sitting again. It was all, I felt, added incentive for her to succeed, not only in the exercises which Miss R endlessly put her to, but most particularly in regaining control over her 'waterworks', lack of which was the biggest obstacle to her homecoming.

We began to live again, in the ordinary ways of life. I remember that only a week or so before, I had seen people sitting on the terrace next to the canteen, drinking a cup of tea or eating an ice cream – other people "laughing"... "drinking"... "planning tomorrow's picnic". But I saw them as through a sheet of plate glass, and it was almost unthinkable that Mary and I might one day sit there ourselves, "laughing" and "drinking", though certainly not "planning tomorrow's picnic". A cup of tea on a hospital canteen patio was my idea of heaven then – I didn't need to look for anything beyond.

And that Tuesday, suddenly and so unexpectedly whisked away to Paradise, we sat and sipped our tea, straight from a hospital urn.

There were very little further foretastes of Paradise during the next fortnight. Miss R's activities were stepped up into overdrive, and the sergeant-majorly aspects of her approach mentioned by that other patient were soon in evidence. Seemingly quite ruthless, in a half-hour session she would typically get Mary upstanding from a bed, walk her with her frame, sit her down again, getting her off one chair and onto a commode, onto the bed again, laying her down on it, sitting her up again, getting her walking straight from the bed, and so on, and so on, with only just time for a breath in between. The seeming ruthlessness was nothing more (or less) than a technique for injecting her patients with some of her own limitless energy and determination; and it worked, session after session, with Mary.

Come to think of it, there was one further taste of Elysium for us, the tailpiece to one of Miss R's blitzkriegs on Mary. It was one of the occasions when I had been required to practise getting Mary into the car. There was nothing special about it: we were getting quite good at it, and earned what was fast becoming Miss R's routine approval. The only difference was that, acting on a sudden impulse, I walked round the car, climbed into the driving seat, and took Mary for a little run round the neighbouring lanes. What a milestone that was!

It wasn't all steady progress that fortnight, under the quasi-military discipline. Again and again when I was with Mary, I carried out my allotted task of single-handedly (behind drawn curtains!) getting her onto the commode, and trying to get her to respond. I well remember one such occasion, when the curtains were parted by the young Mauritian nurse, as I was trying to cope with yet another disappointment. He saw my downhearted look.

"Please don't feel like that about it, she's getting on so well." It was very necessary medicine for me at that moment, and how sensitively he administered it.

Eventually, the problem became the crucial one in regard to Mary's homecoming, and the preoccupation of everyone concerned with her. I remember one day Sister telling me that they were trying a new drug on Mary, and there was a whiff of desperation in the way she said it. But I reminded myself that it was only seven weeks to the day that Mary had been admitted to hospital in a coma, and seven weeks seemed to me early days, for her to recover such subtle control.

It was just then that the social worker chose to add her contribution to the prevailing pessimism by saying that without a catheter it was going to be a formidable laundry problem. A day or two later, and she asked to see me formally.

She was actually a quarter of an hour late for the appointment, and

I waited with considerable apprehension. When she did arrive, she sat me down opposite her, and across the desk top and without any preamble, she fired her opening question at me in a hard-edged, overproduced Oxford accent.

"Are you *determined* to have your wife home, Dr Kemp?"

"I am completely nonplussed by your question," I replied.

And hours later, I still was. Then, with catastrophic suddenness, it came to me that what she had really been hinting at was that it would be better to institutionalise Mary, the euphemism they used which actually meant, "to leave her in hospital for the rest of her life, with me continuing just to visit her, rather than taking responsibility for her again, myself". What a preposterous idea...

Luckily for me, Peggy rang up, and she put a quite different gloss on it, suggesting that the social worker had simply been testing me out, to make sure that I knew what I would be undertaking, especially with the complication of incontinence, if that should continue indefinitely.

In that case, I had left the social worker in no doubt whatever about my determination to have Mary home just as soon as Dr W gave the go-ahead. She had certainly done her best to shake that determination, going on to say, as she had, that it was I they were concerned about, as though all that mattered was that, with Mary 'institutionalised', I could then resume 'normal' life again. Just what kind of person did she think I was?

There was the episode of Mary's swollen left leg, too, which fortunately had a funny side to it. I had noticed during her trips round the grounds in the wheelchair that it had become a little swollen, but one day it was suddenly considerably worse. I mentioned it to Sister when the nurses were getting Mary ready for bed that night.

She looked thoughtful: "Well – it's possible that if it had been both legs, it might have been her kidneys, but as it's only one leg, maybe we've been walking her too much. I didn't let them walk her today," she added.

With some temerity I suggested they might make her leg horizontal in the wheelchair for a while. But she said that maybe it would be better for her to rest in bed for a day; and she found a doctor, who agreed.

The whole thing might have taken on a sombre aspect for me, had it not been for the hilarious time that followed, with the bed – Sister, two nurses, and myself, all trying to find out how to raise the foot of it by means of the mechanism underneath. After quite a number of fruitless and frustrating minutes we realised that we had simply to turn the bed head to foot – it had been installed the wrong way round in the first place!

The next day I took over some coffee-walnut torte, the product of a cooking session I had had the previous day. When Sister saw it she said, with a twinkle in her eye, "So you are practical after all. I had begun to think last night, when you were struggling with the bed, that like most of the doctors round this place you weren't, in spite of your scientific background."

Mary's leg had gone down very nicely, and they seemed well satisfied with it; the postscript from the doctor was that a day or two in bed every so often, was not a bad idea at all, for all of us.

But there was no forgetting the main obstacle to Mary's homecoming. That night, just before I left, they got Mary out of bed, and were obviously despondent to find that she was already wet. I said I would wait, to help get her back into bed again (it was no easy matter), and Sister showed up in the middle of this. Mary had only her slippers on, and therefore had no caliper, so she was obviously very nervous about standing. When, finally, I left, I put my head round Sister's door. Her first comment was that she hadn't yet had a piece of the torte, and I said I hoped she would enjoy it when she did. Suddenly, and seriously then, she asked, "Have you got anyone at home to help you get your wife on and off the bed?" – a question obviously prompted by what she had witnessed earlier.

For the moment, thrown by the remark, I said simply, ingenuously, "No, of course not," but sensing what lay behind her question I added immediately that I had assumed that when three or four weeks thence had been mooted as a possible homecoming time, they had taken into their reckoning the fact that we lived on our own. I did say, too, that if Mary continued to make the kind of progress in the next three or four weeks that she had made in the last ten days, circumstances could be very different then. I was clutching at straws again.

Sister tried to be encouraging about it, but was shrugging her shoulders from time to time, clearly not convinced.

It was late when I finally got back, and her loaded question came home to roost, as I faced myself again, and the whole matter of Mary's homecoming, in the empty house. Doubt reared its ugly head again: perhaps the suggestion of a homecoming three or four weeks thence had not been a fully considered one? Perhaps they hadn't taken into account all the circumstances, after all? I began to wonder, too, what the result of the ward round the next day would be, when all these issues would come up again, including Mary's continued incontinence.

How could I have guessed just how momentous that ward round was to prove?

Chapter Nine

I drove into work very early, and was there soon after 7 o'clock. I left again about 11.30, and drove straight past our home to the Unit. It was about 12.30pm when I arrived. As I passed the open door of Sister's office, I could see Dr W apparently in close conclave with Sister and the social worker; and when Mary was finally ready to be taken out, we had to pass the open door again, to find the conference still going on. I said "Hello" to Dr W who, just then, did nothing more than acknowledge it. But Mary and I had hardly settled in our favourite spot on the canteen terrace when out they came, all three of them.

At once, I was called over; and again one of those near-photographic images that the mind stows away on momentous occasions comes back to me so vividly – of Mary sitting apart from us, in her wheelchair, looking so far away (though it was only a matter of yards) and so vulnerable, as we embarked on nothing less than settling her future, among the four of us. What fearsome responsibilities we sometimes have for the fate of others, and how fortunate perhaps it is, that, at the time, we are oblivious of it....

It was the social worker, in fact, who started the ball rolling by putting me in the witness box (or was it the dock?), and proceeding to cross-examine me all over again about the seriousness of my intent to have Mary home, and the extent of my awareness of all the difficulties that would be involved. What did it take to persuade the woman that I was serious – more than that, that I was totally committed to having Mary home? But I suspect, actually, that it was some sort of replay for Dr W's benefit.

Poor Mary – as she sat there, so quietly, just out of earshot. I looked across at her, and wondered what was going through her mind. I couldn't tell, for the wheelchair was facing partly away from us, and I couldn't even wave to her, to reassure her. It was this awesome passivity of hers. No, that's the wrong word, for it might suggest unthinking inactivity. It was positive acceptance of all that life did to her, indeed, of all that life threw at her, so often bringing something truly life-enhancing out of what might have been deemed unmitigated evil. I was never more conscious than in that moment, of my responsibilities to her – to provide her, as far as it was possible, with yet another lease of life in which she could bestow upon family and friends alike that giveaway love of hers.

Dr W took over then, reminding me that when we had first met he had told me that he would always be straight with me. So, he said, he must tell me now that he wasn't able to say exactly how full Mary's recovery would be from the damage that the stroke had done. But he went on then to say that he believed our "mutual devotion", as he put it, was going to stand us in good stead. Provided, therefore, that I could "pick up the tricks of the trade" from Miss R to enable me to manage Mary on my own, there was no reason why she shouldn't come home almost immediately.

I was dumbfounded, but the social worker had left us by then, and I seized the opportunity to quiz him about her blunt, unadorned question that had hit me so hard, and was still rankling: "Are you still determined to have your wife home?"

"That was a straightforward enough question, surely?" he responded.

"Are you really implying that I should contemplate Mary becoming institutionalised?"

He said, "That was surely something you would have had to consider during these past weeks?"

Momentarily I faltered. "I can barely contemplate it," I stammered, adding then, immediately, "in fact, I cannot contemplate it, certainly not at this juncture, and perhaps never."

That settled it – I had finally convinced them, and from then on they seemed to come right over to my side, and began to discuss practicalities, and the whole mechanics of Mary's homecoming.

Dr W left then, and Sister deliberately hung behind, and gave me a wonderful pep talk. She said how she hated catheters, and that she believed that with a washing machine and tumble drier I would be able to cope with the incontinence problem very satisfactorily. She went on to say that she thought it was by far the best thing for Mary to come home, and that she believed that Mary would make "really good progress" at home, and that the two of us together would in fact "make a go of it." Professional non-involvement had been thrown to the winds, as her face shone with a shared joy, and her voice, quite apart from the words she was using, conveyed the tremendous warmth of her encouragement.

As things turned out, Mary spent only ten more days in the Unit, and they can only be described as days of creative chaos. I am sure that the chaos was apparent rather than real. It was this 'sleight of hand' thing that Willow Ward was so good at – in fact, one might be tempted to think that the ward provided a classic example of the so-called 'chaos theory', where a small, and almost imperceptible change produces a large-scale outcome!

There were an increasing number of sessions with Miss R for both Mary and me; and I had to open up a second front at home. There was the elimination of rugs, and the laying of carpet tiles where necessary. There was the reorganisation of the tiny kitchen, so that it could accommodate a washing machine and tumble drier, which meant major surgery on the kitchen units and cupboards; and there were appointments to keep with tradesmen, particularly the plumber, so that the whole house, with its functional face-lift, could successfully spring into action the instant Mary was home again. And, as a foretaste of that for Mary, during one of our afternoon trips in the car I took her right past the end of our road.

My efforts to make her aware again of signals from her 'waterworks' were greatly intensified, too, in those last ten days, and began to produce results, literally as well as metaphorically, and to our mutual joy. And let it be said that few joys, can be more basic, or more satisfying, than such a one!

Even the social worker, whom I still felt had handled me so rawly, seemed to suffer a sea change. I met her one day as I was leaving the Unit. Abruptness seemed to be her style, for she hove to, and asked baldly, how soon could I resign my job?

I said, "In a matter of days."

She responded, "Well, you'd better do so here and now, because after the next ward round I think we shall be advising that your wife comes home, as early as it can be arranged."

The next day I sought an interview at work to discuss the matter, only to discover to my great relief that they had already been considering the situation, anticipating that there would be the need for an immediate change. I was overwhelmed by the extent of their understanding and sympathy. They had, as one possibility, been contemplating changing my status to that of a consultant, and, as another, an informal arrangement in which my job (already reduced to a part-time one before Mary had had the second stroke) would be done for the most part at home (after all, the bulk of it was paper work).

I discussed with my scientist colleague all that would be involved in the transitional period following Mary's homecoming, and the fact that, in the battle for Mary, we had even persuaded the social worker to change sides. I went on to say that, as a scientist, I was unorthodox enough to believe that in these situations there were imponderables – inscrutable elements – at work, which depended on aspects of life and being which are indeed unfathomable to science: they couldn't be measured, and they couldn't be weighed – they had, by their very nature, a quality of singularity which meant that they couldn't be tested endlessly for repeatability under predetermined conditions. Yet, I argued, they were of inestimable importance, adding for good measure that I believed that Mary and I together, and especially in our own home, could call these imponderable resources into play. Of course I had an axe to grind – but it was an axe which I believed in with my whole being.

My colleague smiled at me indulgently, that I should have assumed that he would take a great deal of persuading to agree with me.

Quietly, he said that there was no need for me to argue my case: he fully agreed ("in a gentle sort of way," as he put it) with all I had said. What a difference it was to make in the weeks and months that were to follow, to know that in the particular scientific fraternity where I lived and moved and had my professional being there was such understanding of the nature of the terrain into which Mary and I would be venturing together.

Nevertheless, even as I write, I have been reminded all too plainly of the existence of a subspecies within the ranks of my fellow-scientists that treats what he would regard as the 'arrogance of belief' with what can only be described as an equal 'arrogance of disbelief'. Just minutes ago, one such was pontificating on the radio about the way in which the 'scientific culture' had swept aside 'once and for all' [sic] the 'religious culture'. And to make sure that his listeners were aware that he knew exactly what mumbo-jumbo the latter comprised, he cited the (hypothetical) case of an imam who might be observed saying to members of his sect, "I shall drop this fork three times, and the third time, instead of falling to the table, it will rise to the ceiling." (Those were, substantively, his actual words.)

The programme was a debate marking the fact that the British Association for the Advancement of Science was meeting that week. It did make me wonder how far some of my fellow scientists had really advanced after all, in the understanding, not of the mechanics of life, but of its meaning.

After the discussion about the future of my job, there was a tremendous sense of the decks having at last been cleared for action – and there was plenty of action in those few days that remained.

At the end of it all, practically everything that could be done to make the house safe for Mary had been done, and the 'functional face-lift' that was to make it as efficient as possible for me to run, and as safe as possible for Mary to live in, was more or less complete. The commode, with its seat lovingly padded by Miss R, was installed in the bedroom, the 'Stand Easy' was standing at ease by the bed, awaiting Mary's arrival, and the plumber had finally plumbed in the washing machine, grafted, like a major surgical transplant, into one of the kitchen units; whilst the kitchen cabinet (would 'Hygena' ever forgive me for it?) had been 'cannibalised' to take the tumble drier, the 4-inch exhaust ducting of which had been made to wend its leisurely way through the larder and out into the back porch.

A night or two before Mary came home I gave the washing machine its chance to show its paces, congratulating myself on the transformation the kitchen had undergone, as I lay in bed listening to the machine bowling round with its first bundle of towels. I felt quite smug about it, really – that is, until the morning, when I found that I'd failed to put in the washing powder.

We were actually into those last few days, too, before I was finally able to report to Sister some real success with what had for so long been known as the 'waterworks problem'. She said, so generously, "Well, you were right, weren't you? – you were right!", and she went on to affirm once again her strong dislike and distrust of catheters.

It was all hustle and bustle on Mary's behalf, and two young nurses, endeavouring to put her through her paces as they got her into bed one night, were addressed archly, by Mary, after she had giggled her way through most of the proceedings. "If you're going to treat me like that I think I'd better go to another hospital!"

This earned the instant riposte from one of the nurses, "Don't you worry, you'll get treated the same, wherever you are!"

It produced a laugh all round, but how true it was – in an unintentional way. For such was Mary's nature that even if a relationship had started off as a casual one, in one way or another it inevitably ended up as something special.

I had, as usual, spent Mary's lunchtime with her. First, then, the social worker had a word with me, followed directly after by Dr W.

He began in a matter-of-fact tone of voice, as though he was deliberately trying to hold himself back. "Well, we shall be sending your wife home now in a day or two." Then, suddenly, as though he could restrain himself no longer, and almost blurting it out, he added, "You know, your wife has done wonderfully well."

He went on to say that they would like to follow her up, and asked if I would take her regularly to the Day Hospital at the Unit; it would ensure her continued progress, he said, and it would be a help to me too, by giving me a few hours off, regularly. His parting shot was to say that there was no reason why Mary should not recover to a "near-normal" life again; and with what was undoubtedly more than a touch of hyperbole he added, "We'll have her shopping in town on her own yet, and then she can buy me a pint!"

He had said enough now for it to be obvious that he had been profoundly impressed – even deeply moved – by all that had transpired during that one brief month since he had admitted Mary to his Unit: there is no denying that it had been little short of a miracle. But, alas, Mary was destined never to go shopping again – never to go anywhere on her own again. And she was never to buy Dr W his pint of beer.

Just as he was preparing to leave us Mary suddenly said to him, "Do have a good holiday, won't you?"

He realised that the fact that he was going on holiday had stayed in her memory for the whole hour that he had been with us, and with real astonishment he turned to the social worker and said, "Do you see now what I mean?"

I couldn't help wondering whether he, too, had had to do battle with her scepticism.

Mary spent her last day in the Unit quietly confident, no doubt borne up by the knowledge that the next day she would be in her own home again, having spent two months in hospital, to the day.

My last memory of that stay was of the final evening, when I turned up at supper time with a copy of *Wireless World*, which I had treated myself to, for the first time for a very long while.

Mary spotted it at once, and then, looking me straight in the eye, she said, "Gosh! You must be feeling better!"

She was right, too! – I was on Cloud Nine.

I had done a lot towards her homecoming, but nothing like all I had hoped and intended to do. But I could afford to be a little philosophical about it now; for, after all, what hadn't already been done would be done now in Mary's company. Surely it was rare for procrastination to be rewarded – and so richly.

> Now you are coming home,
> My love –
> Home to us all!
> Yet, were truth better served
> To say that home
> Is coming back to us –
> For you are home!
> Bricks and mortar
> Have ever been
> Merely the place
> For you to be
> What you are:
> Wife,
> Mother,
> Friend of all!
> So!
> Sing bricks!
> Sing mortar!
> And sing, my darling daughter!
> Rejoice, my sons!
> For home is coming back
> To each and all
> Of us.

Chapter Ten

It was late evening, on Sunday, August 28th, the end of four hectic and at times tumultuous days – Mary's first four days back home. There hadn't been a single moment in which I could sit down and add even a word to the tape diary: and until that moment I had even forgotten that August 28th was our little grandson's first birthday. Our son John and daughter-in-law Catherine had arrived from Canterbury to give us some moral support for a few days, and at long last I had a chance to sit down quietly by myself to recollect and to record the more memorable moments of those unforgettable days.

It is not in the least surprising that what came instantly to mind was an incident which in retrospect was very funny indeed, though whilst it was happening it was quite otherwise.

It concerned Mary's very first use of the commode, lovingly refurbished by Miss R. To my horror, Mary's 'sit-upon' had apparently developed the most appalling water blisters within the first few hours of her being home again. I was petrified. How could I confess to Sister that I had so grossly mismanaged things as to have caused Mary to come out in such awful blisters (they were three or four millimetres across, and nearly hemispherical) within an hour or two of having her home?

I re-examined the evidence closely, still absolutely horrified. Suddenly, and to my enormous relief, I realised then that the 'blisters' were in fact, quite regularly spaced, and that what I was looking at was, literally, an impression of the perforations in the plastic padding which Miss R had added to the seat....

But the best moment of all, of those first four days, had been earlier that evening, very soon after putting Mary to bed. The way I had been shown to do this meant that she inevitably ended up on her back, and that is how I had left her. A little later, I pushed the bedroom door open noiselessly to see how she was getting on; and there she was, sound asleep, curled up, with her back towards me. Despite all the fear of rolling over that she had shown in hospital, she had turned over of her own accord.

That was, and has remained, one of the most wonderful moments of my life: the first fruits of her homecoming – for her to have lost such a basic fear, just like that, and to have her tucked up and sound asleep in her own bed again, for the first time for nine weeks, and looking so very snug! There was that moment too, on the second night. I had forgotten to brush her teeth (something which she was never again going to be able to do for herself). She was already tucked up in bed when I remembered it, and I said, "Sorry, I'll have to come back to do your teeth."

"Right!" she said, with a roguish grin, "And when you do, I'll open my mouth for you."

Then, as I finally tucked her up, I was suddenly overwhelmed by the simple affection she had always shown to all and sundry, and found myself saying to her, "You've loved so many people, so much, haven't you?"

She said, quaintly, "Not quite!" Her little difficulty with words could be very endearing sometimes.

When one has been anticipating so keenly such a momentous event as Mary's homecoming, one rightly thinks only of the joy involved, discounting the difficulties – many of them grave – that one knows it must bring in its wake. How otherwise, would any such dream ever become reality?

How near to being unrealisable our particular dream was, is to be gauged by the fact that in my parting exchanges with Sister she had said, quietly and soberly, that they would be keeping Mary's place in the ward open for two weeks. If such a remark had come from some of the other professionals with whom I had had to deal during the course of Mary's illnesses (the "what your wife needs is a new set of arteries" brigade) it would simply have angered me. But by then I knew Sister well enough to believe that she was on the side of the angels; and on my side too, in my determination to have Mary home again, and that her offer stemmed straightforwardly from her assessment of the nature and extent of the difficulties we were facing. But the image of that empty bed waiting for Mary to return to it simply spurred me on, to make sure that as soon as possible it would be allocated to the next patient waiting for the wonders of Willow Ward to be worked upon her.

The joy enshrined in the mental images of those first few days of Mary's homecoming (and so sharply recorded and vividly retained in my mind's eye) was indeed real and deep. But, inevitably, it soon became clouded by the need to acknowledge, at least to myself, that the task we had undertaken was, indeed, a herculean one. Once more I was having to admit to myself the stark difference between dealing with Mary in the ward, under the beady eye of Miss R, or Sister, or one the ward staff, and having to cope alone, with no second or third line of defence to fall back on. There was a sense in which I had staked our whole future on our being able to manage, and the stakes were being called in so quickly it seemed.

Thus it was only a matter of a day or two before the problem of ever being able to get Mary down the front steps of the house and into the car loomed ominously. There were seven or eight steps, wide and sloping, and, as yet, no handrail (something else I had overlooked). To get some idea of the problem John and I put a 56lb weight (nothing like Mary's weight, though!) into the wheelchair and tried taking it up and down to the road. It didn't take us long to reach the conclusion that it would be utterly impossible for one person to cope, unaided. Then we had the bright idea of asking our neighbours (who occupied the other one of the semidetached pair) if we could make a gap in the hedge dividing the two front gardens so that I could take Mary straight along the front of the two houses, and then down the neighbour's path to the pavement (the road itself was a hill, and the next-door house, being further up the hill, had no need of a flight of steps – just a single one to the pavement). There was, I sensed, a momentary but understandable hesitation (an Englishman's home is, after all, his castle) but I am sure that immediately afterwards they felt that it would be a piece of good neighbourliness which would bring us closer together. But a few days later this arrangement very nearly led to disaster.

In the meantime, our main preoccupation during those first few days was Mary's walking. In particular, there was great difficulty in getting her to walk without the frame: she would regularly manage just a few steps only, and we would have to give up. Often, instructions just seemed to muddle her – but where could one get to, without instructions? It soon began to be very frustrating.

Then, one evening, acting on a sudden inspiration, I tried incentive instead. She was sitting in a chair which gave her rather a limited view of the television, and I simply pointed to another chair across the room and said, "I think that would be a better chair for television, don't you?"

She agreed straightaway, so I said, without further comment or instructions, "Come on then, let's go."

I offered her my arm, and she stood up and walked, just like that!

When it was bedtime, we repeated the sequence. I said, "Do you want to go to bed now?"

She said she did, so once again, I responded, quite simply, with "Come on! Let's go then!" And away we went.

It would have been easy to think then that we had 'cracked it', as they say, but it was by no means so: it continued to be as much a matter of confidence as anything else, and this applied to the caliper too. One might have thought that the caliper was actually essential, but it had never been proven so, and there were times when Mary would walk perfectly well without it. In consequence, alas, both the walking frame and the caliper were in danger of becoming bones of contention between us, and the honeymoon period of Mary's homecoming soon threatened to become a battle of wills.

There was one memorable day when, after a tremendous struggle (poor Mary!), I had to give in, and put the caliper back on again, as well as letting her have the walking frame back. How harsh it seems now, in retrospect – but I still believe that that bit of 'stiffening' was necessary (had some of Miss R's approach rubbed off on me?).

Anyway, later that day I adopted different tactics to work our way back. First, without any argument or debate, I put the caliper on, and offered Mary the walking frame, to get her feeling relaxed again about walking. Then, again without any discussion at all, I casually changed her calipered shoes for the ordinary ones, but left her with the walking frame, which she went off with, quite happily. Then we quietly discarded the walking frame, and to my great satisfaction she found that she could walk without the frame, and in ordinary shoes.

Once rid of the frame, Mary would walk behind me in the manner of a slow Conga dance, as we had been taught by Miss R, but after a few days this also didn't seem to be effective any more. It was then that I suggested she tried simply walking on my arm. Wearing her calipered shoes, she did this quite successfully, and the next day, without comment, I put her ordinary shoes on, and again she set off on my arm, this time down the garden – halfway down and back again in fact, just with her arm lightly tucked into mine!

Later still that day, she walked about the house simply holding my hand beside her, and then, on at least a couple of occasions, she walked two or three yards towards me entirely on her own. There was a sort of aura about such happenings – dare I say it? – the aura almost of miracle. Not because they were miraculous, but because they came about, often unexpectedly, and seemingly against great odds. It certainly wasn't because I had any special powers either: anyone could have done the same. All that was required was to convince Mary that you believed that she could do it.

So, day by day we lived and learned – certainly that it was not always best to make a frontal attack on a problem, nor for that matter, for me simply to role-play the sergeant-major. Anyway, as far as I was concerned, that was completely out of character!

It was not all a teeth-gritting, pressing-on-regardless sort of existence – there were often moments of comic relief, when we could have a little giggle about something that had happened, or even about ourselves! The fact that I was new to such things as washing machines and tumble driers regularly showed up. There were still occasions when we ended up with a beautifully rinsed but unwashed batch of clothes, as a result of my having forgotten the washing powder yet again. And there was the day when paper pads got as far as the tumble drier, where they disintegrated, and the remnants wedged themselves between the rotating drum and the casing of the machine, bringing the whole thing to a standstill, and blowing the fuse.

There was the matter of the spinning wheel too, which, bearing in mind the deadly earnest nature of much of our existence, added almost a fairy tale touch.

We had our friend Marie to tea. She had a spinning wheel, and brought samples of the wool she was spinning, and we quickly homed onto the idea that treadling might be a much more enjoyable form of physiotherapy for Mary's right foot and leg than the more formal and technical exercises. At least, it might constitute something more in the nature of occupational therapy, and perhaps even have an end product! So we arranged to go round to inspect the spinning wheel, and have Mary try it out, which we duly did a few days later. The upshot of all this was that a spinning wheel kit was ordered, and its assembly, and commissioning, was something which I looked forward to very much, as a piece of occupational therapy for myself.

Life was laced, and lightened too, with the little quips that Mary continually came out with, often made all the more delightful by the quaint twist they would be given by her difficulties at times with the choice of words.

There was the occasion when I was discussing with her the fact that she didn't fret at all about herself, and that I felt that that was one of the things that was helping her to make such good progress. She replied, quite simply, "I suppose I like things as they are." What she really meant, I am sure, was that she took things as they were. But what a succinct way of putting it! – and I'm sure that that was one of Mary's great secrets.

She showed great high spirits too, sometimes at the end of a busy and often trying day for her. I remember very well indeed one evening when she was sitting looking more than a little tired, and I asked her if she was ready for bed.

"Oh! I don't know about that," she said promptly, "as a matter of fact I was just wondering if you would like to come and cuddle me." And when she did finally set off for bed she said she would like to call in at the loo, "That is, if you happen to be going that way," she added.

It is difficult to convey the quality of her mood when she produced these little gems of repartee. It was as though – how shall I put it? – as though she was savouring every nuance of the delicate and delicious flavour of her involvement again in the little everyday things of life, with the 'palate' that only those who have been very near to death acquire.

There was a moment, only four days after she had come home, when an error of judgement on my part – or, perhaps to be kinder to myself, a lack of experience – brought her close again if not to death, then at least to serious injury.

Isobel, a frail and elderly friend of ours, had been to tea, and with a modest amount of purely moral support from her, something possessed me to try out our new route to the pavement and the waiting car, via our neighbour's front garden. I knew that Mary weighed at least three times as much as the 56lb weight which John and I had used in our experiments, but then, we weren't going down those awful front steps of ours, and the route to the single step at our neighbour's front gate was a very gentle slope, and child's play by comparison.

What I didn't realise was that with a wheelchair it was much wiser to go down a step backwards, which gives you much better control of the weight, as the wheelchair negotiates the step. Instead, without a thought, I pushed the chair straight over the edge until its rear wheels were suddenly suspended in mid-air over the lip of the step. At that moment the whole weight of Mary and the chair all but snatched the handles out of my hands, as I fought to hang on there were fierce pins and needles all round my neck and shoulders, as desperately taut muscles pressed down on tortured nerves. It was a terrible moment, for if I had lost my grip Mary and the chair would have gone careering down the road (which was a steep hill) and all the achievements of the previous two months would have been brought to a sudden end – or so it seemed to me at that moment. But it was a lesson I needed to learn only once; and that night I had a long, hot soak in the bath, to try to ease my aching shoulders and haunches.

Exactly one week after Mary came home, I wrote to Dr W. The letter was yet another milestone, written in the first flush of the joy of having Mary home again, and with a continued reluctance to admit that it was a mountain face and not an alpine meadow that lay ahead of us:

"Today I took Mary to the Day Hospital for the first time...

"What a memorable day it has been! ...We were received like old friends...

"What a transformation since I made that phone call to you at 10 o'clock at night only six weeks ago ... In view of what I now know about Willow Ward I realise the extent of your forbearance that night...

"I cannot possibly say what it has all amounted to for me...

"Suffice it to say that the greatest mental suffering I have ever experienced was transformed into something positive and creative, instead of my being crushed by it."

Chapter Eleven

That letter was dated September 1st, 1977; and four days ago, and 14 years on, it was September 1st again. I said to a friend that the clerk of the weather seemed to be well aware of the date, for August 31st had been a hot summer's day, and then, overnight, the temperature had fallen dramatically, and the mists were upon us again – now, as then, "casting their immemorial spell". But 14 years ago it was not just a hint of autumn in the air that had sobered my mood.

We had a visit from our GP – his first since Mary's homecoming, and something prompted me to take the lid off some of my pent-up fears and apprehensions, which up to that moment I had hardly been prepared to admit, even to myself.

He had asked me how Mary had been, generally, and it was then that I had referred to the euphoria again, which on occasion was worrying me stiff. For the first time he started talking of "a little frontal lobe damage". In the state of mind I was in, that seemed an unbearably harsh way of putting it, although it was all in a day's work, so to say, for him. Actually, he was a good doctor, and a very good friend to us, but I had had a surfeit of that sort of purely technical comment over the years – "what your wife needs is a new set of arteries" the classic example, which I still had only to think of to be overwhelmed all over again by a sense of helplessness and near-hopelessness.

It can be argued that in the busy life of a doctor there is no time to pick one's words; yet if one such remark had doused my faith in Mary's ability to recover – my faith, the faith of the one destined to be her 'companion in the way' in the long haul back to health – what an incalculable loss that would have been to Mary, and, indeed, to the forces which the doctor himself was presumably attempting to muster on her behalf. Or did he discount any such contribution of mine alongside the 16-inch guns of modern drugs lined up for her? The drugs certainly had their place, but so did the faith in Mary of those who loved her dearly; and to do anything, however unwittingly, to undermine that was surely, at the lowest estimate, a grave tactical error in the battle for Mary's restoration to health.

Whatever the case, for the time being I had suffered more than enough from such pronouncements. So far as the euphoria was concerned, I suppose that, despite my fears, I still believed deep down that it might well go away, as Mary felt more confident and more secure, and realised that her daily life amongst family and friends was being restored to her again. Meanwhile, as Gerard Manley Hopkins put it, I needed to "christen my wild-worst best."

A kind of claustrophobia was creeping in too – about not being able to get out of the house at all, except to go just beyond the back door, to the dustbin. And that evening, following our doctor's visit, when I did just that, I found that the stars were out; and I gazed at the autumn sky, and longed to be looking at it with Mary, and to be free to walk with her in the evening time again. And I realised how many years it actually was, since we had walked together in the dusk, or in the dark. I had to pull myself up sharply then, and to remind myself of the miracle it was just to have her home again, as well and as mobile as she was, and of the need to stop dwelling on what might have been and now could never be.

But it wasn't easy to dismiss such ideas from one's head, or such feelings from one's heart, just like that. These were no mere skirmishes with the occasional defecting thought or the momentary traitorous feeling; they were battles, wars of attrition, that went on, day on day, and night on night, threatening the very supply lines of physical strength and spiritual energy I needed in the fight to restore Mary's health, and to gain a new span of life for her.

It was like being sniped at from all directions. One day it would be the sheer weight of household chores, and on another it would be a single moment of nostalgia that would be my undoing, when I would come suddenly and unexpectedly upon something in the house which would be so devastatingly evocative of the past, and of "joy which I scarce now dare contemplate." The 'claustrophobia' would take strange inverted forms – for example, a horror of the sense of separation and cut-off-ness which our circumstances inevitably produced. There was, for instance, an airmail letter one morning from friends in Australia, and as I picked it up off the mat sheer panic overwhelmed me for a moment, at the thought that 10000 miles – yes, ten thousand seemingly unbridgeable miles – lay between them and us.

There was a dire need to accept what Tielhard de Chardin would have called the "diminishments" involved in what had happened to us, and to look forwards, and not backwards, or even sideways. In Harry Williams' words, "It hurts when the manacles which chain us to the past are broken. And it hurts when by our experience we are opened up almost forcibly to [a new] future. It seems like one single hurt, leaving us all too agonisingly aware of its destructive power and almost totally unaware of its creative power, save for the faint glimmer of undefined hope."

Yet "diminishments" have their compensations, too. As some of the more conventional pleasures and satisfactions of life are scaled down or even phased out, what one has tended to look upon as the incidental or even insignificant ones assume their rightful place again in the order of things, from which they had long since been demoted. Thus, I remember baking bread one night just as something to do. But its role and function went far beyond that. Man has been making bread for thousands of years, and I believe that the very rhythm of kneading the dough evokes folk memories which tend to re-establish within us the very roots of our humanity. Fanciful? Not a bit of it – try it one day.

Anyway, it doesn't stop at making the bread: I knew how Mary's eyes would light up next morning when I took her breakfast, and announced, "Chef's compliments, and it's home-made bread this morning!" I am sure that it literally 'did her good' – that this relishing of simple and wholesome things is all too rare these days of convenience foods, and has real therapeutic value, literally and metaphorically restoring a 'taste' for life and living in all their aspects.

Just over a fortnight after Mary's homecoming we were invited back to a party in Willow Ward, and culinary activities came into their own again. It was to be on Sunday September 11th, and the night before, after getting Mary to bed, I spent making a batch of chocolate eclairs, and some spicy Turkish coffee-walnut squares (my own particular 'flavour of the month'). The weather forecast was good, and although it was still a great adventure taking Mary out in the car, there was every prospect that we should make it. Indeed, in the event, Mary walked all the way from the car to the ward, and then, with discretion the better part of valour, she had a wheelchair to the far end, where all the 'goodies' were set out.

There was nothing special to celebrate. The ward parties were apparently a regular though not all that frequent event, intended to break down the formal image of the hospital (as if that weren't being done all the time in Willow Ward) and to provide a touch of the homely and domestic, with the longer-stay patients particularly in mind. It was another of those 'extra miles' that the ward was prepared to go, part of the tender loving care which was the backbone of the more conventional therapy that was the basis of their working day.

Typically, though, it didn't meet with the unqualified approval of the Sister on duty that Sunday. She had a heart of gold, but was very down-to-earth, straight and to the point in her language. I looked round at the sumptuous spread of sandwiches and cakes and bowls of trifle and the like, and facetiously remarked to her that it looked as though they might need a few indigestion tablets by the end of the proceedings. The response was prompt and characteristic. She said that although she had actually organised the party, it had been under some duress. Waving her hand down the ward she said that they were overfed (she was probably right about that), going on to say that the food ought really to have been taken out to all those old folk who were living alone, and who "hardly ever saw any good food", as she put it. She added (with a slightly confessional air) that in view of this she expected the staff would have at least some of my cakes.

When I replied that that had certainly been the intention anyway, she murmured, "Oh, thanks very much!" as though that had salved her conscience!

I am convinced that with Mary there was a tendency for normality to breed more normality. Thus, after that bit of normal life and living at the party, and faced with the open door of the car, she just put her right foot in first, sat down, and then drew her left leg in after her (just as she had always done). No clumsy manoeuvre any more on my part, to get her back round towards the car, bottom in first then, and head down, lifting her feet in last. All that had gone, not by taking careful thought, or as the result of a lot of practice, but simply by 'losing herself' in the ward party, and then 'finding herself' responding to the stimulus of the open car door in the time-honoured way. Another cautionary tale about taking our problems too seriously, and too often making frontal attacks on them?

A night or two later, when I was putting her to bed, I tried the same technique. Instead of the elaborate rigmarole of telling her to put her hands behind her, and to lift her body, and so on and so on, I simply said, "Put your head down on the pillow now," and she made a very creditable attempt at doing so, without any of the rigmarole.

But the most thrilling instance of this came a day or two later still. Before lunch, I had taken Mary to the dining room and put her in her usual chair to await the arrival of lunch. I went back a minute or two later to find her laying the table. This meant that she had got up from her chair, walked round unaided to the sideboard, got out the cutlery, and taken it back to the table. It was marvellous, little short of miraculous really. But (Oh, ye of little faith!) I found myself ticking her off, albeit good-naturedly, and pointing out the very real risks she had been taking.

How does one strike a balance between encouragement and necessary caution? I didn't know then, and I still don't think I know, even now. But there was no doubt at all about the fact that slowly but surely the home surroundings were drawing out of Mary all the old actions and responses, just as I had hoped and believed they would.

And she was talking too, about repotting all the houseplants! Just think that I might have been persuaded to allow her to be 'institutionalised'...

It was not simply a case of Mary gritting her teeth and tackling her problems with grim determination, either: she continually showed flashes of her old, skittish sense of humour.

Thus, following her initiative at laying the table, that same night when I was putting her to bed I had to leave her sitting on the side of it, whilst I went back into the kitchen to sort something out that needed my attention. When I got back she was lying snugly tucked up in bed, looking very coy, and with her head just where it should be on the pillow, still a very difficult manoeuvre for her.

I was astonished, and said, "How did you do that?" and she simply said, with a lovely look on her face, "Ah, well, you'll have to wait till next time to find that out, won't you?"

There was the occasion too, when, with the spinning wheel I had ordered all assembled and in action, she had suddenly got the hang of it, and was busy treadling away, and I said to her, "That's very good!" She replied, all in one breath, "Yes-it-is-pretty-good-and-I-shall-want-bread-and-jam-for-my-tea," – for all the world as though she was claiming her reward.

But perhaps the loveliest example of all was provided by the intercom which I had installed between the bedroom and the sitting room. I had had grave doubts as to whether Mary would be able to manage it. I well remember taking her a small transistor radio when she was in Dr W's unit. I had tuned it to Radio 4 and taped down the tuning knob (she would have been quite incapable of the tuning operation at that time), so that all she had to do was to click it "On" and "Off". But it turned out that she was quite unable to do even that at the time.

Things were very different, though, the first night the intercom went into action. She was continually 'buzzing' me, chatting away to me on it, and operating the 'press to talk' button correctly, as though she had been doing it all her life. What a transformation!

A few nights later, after the workmen had been to re-concrete the paths and the front steps, Mary was in bed, and I had been busy for some time, writing, in the sitting-room. Suddenly, the buzzer sounded, and I went to see what she wanted. She said baldly, even a little anxiously (presumably having become aware of the silence), "Are you alright?"

I replied, "Yes, of course I am!", adding facetiously, "Did you think I had fallen down a well or something? – you know I'd come and tell you if I was going to do anything like that."

Not to be outdone, she said drolly, "Oh, well, I thought you might have got stuck in the concrete."

We are back to this matter of laughter and its crucial place in human life and relationships. In retrospect, and bearing in mind the difficulties that Mary experienced so often in finding just the right word after that second stroke, it is clear now that it was when humour took over, and laughter became the vehicle, that all such barriers to communication between us came down again for a few precious moments.

On these occasions the exchanges between us were more like a piece of jocular counterpoint from a Bach duo. Mary would suddenly produce a jolly little 'tune' from somewhere deep down inside her – from that well of humour which she had always possessed, and which had far from run dry: it had just got silted over during the worst of the times she had been through. And it would be a tune that owed nothing to the past, nor borrowed anything from the future – it simply related to the matter of the moment; and sensing this, I would respond to it, and, so to say, at Mary's invitation, briefly, all too briefly, enter into her 'Eternal Now'. And my 'tune' would interweave with hers, and for those few moments time would stand still for us. No – better to say that for a few precious moments we stood outside time.

> Oh! how we met! –
> In a fourth dimension
> (Not of Einstein's time,
> But freed
> Of its constraint
> And tension)....

But there were other and much more sombre themes inside me clamouring to be heard, and which, after all that had happened to Mary, I would never again be able to share with her. Maybe, I should say, "could never again attempt to share with her", for, perhaps, as suggested earlier, she was already living in a world of pure spirit after that second stroke, a world where she had left behind once and for all the cares and worries of lesser mortals.

Take, for instance, the visit of our former vicar, which, in spite of (or was it because of?) his high spirits, precipitated such nostalgia, and finally such sheer, black depression in me; Mary, by contrast, was one of Blake's breed, who

> ... kisses the Joy as it flies,
> Lives in Eternity's sunrise.

Tom was on his way up to the university to give a lecture, and rang to ask if he could call on us. It was only a little after ten in the morning, a rare time to have a visitor, a particularly welcome one at that. The recollection of waking to the harsher realities of another daily round was still very much with me, and the long haul of getting breakfast, and then of washing and dressing Mary and getting her up had only just come to an end when the doorbell rang. Tom was no ordinary visitor, and no ordinary friend. He had shared so many of the crucial times in our lives during the last ten or fifteen years. It was he who had joined me within five minutes of my finding Mary unconscious on the landing in 1968, he who had injected me with the faith that she could and would recover; and it was he who only ten days into Mary's second illness, had expressed the same faith in her powers of recovery. Even as I went to the door I was wondering what was this inside information that Tom had about Mary?

He was certainly not the facile sort who would say such things simply because they cost nothing, or because he thought that that was what you were wanting to hear him say. Not at all. When he spoke of Mary in such terms it was with the same kind of quiet assurance that would be shown by a medical man, who, in possession of all the facts, was prepared to state his conclusions confidently.

With the clearer perspective provided by being fourteen years on, I am quite convinced that Tom was aware of certain qualities in Mary which, from within the daily struggle to cope I was unaware of; that he had a shrewd idea of the place which Mary had come to occupy in the spiritual order of things – that in some respects her spirit was indeed already outside of Einstein's time, and "freed of its constraint and tension", with all the potentiality for healing and wholeness which that brought with it.

I pondered these things as I walked along the hall to open the door. It was a wonderful day, weather-wise, which would seem to complete the blessings and benefits that the day had brought with it. For Mary, it probably did; but for me, with all the perversity of my make-up, the sunshine seemed only to enhance the feeling of isolation which preoccupation with Mary's illness tended to foster ("Here we are with our pain... and for the rest of the world it is business as usual").

Largely confined as we were to the house by the circumstances, that perverse bit of me would start thinking, inter alia, of all the things we might have been doing on a fine day. (We had booked a holiday just before Mary had been taken ill, and but for that we wouldn't even have been there to receive Tom – we would have been drinking in the beauties of the Lake District.) And as for Tom – just because he was the friend he was, always at hand in a crisis – his associations perforce included many sombre ones.

That day Mary went to bed for her afternoon rest more than pleased to have seen Tom again (after all, laughter was a major part of Tom's stock-in-trade), but as for myself, I spent Mary's rest time fighting off black depression again. Ill-advisedly, I had decided on some long-delayed tidying-up, and it wasn't long before I came upon a bureau whose pigeon holes were stuffed full of memorabilia. I ought never to have tackled it, considering the mood I was in already. And working my way through the contents of the bureau, my mood worsened steadily as I stumbled on old photographs, keepsakes and the like, from years and years before.

A couple of months later, and I had to suffer the spectacle of Mary happily going through the selfsame things. I say "suffer", because it was agony simply for me to watch her dwelling (quite unhealthily, so it seemed to me) on the past. It was Peggy who once again came to the rescue, saying that I must be patient with Mary, and pointing out that in all probability it was helping her to re-establish her roots after all that she had been through. What a blessing it is to have not merely friends, but wise ones!

I remember, too, that night after Tom had called. As noted already, our bedroom was downstairs, and had been our dining-room for most of the time we were bringing up our family. I lay in the darkness, with Mary already sound asleep, tracing the hazy outline of the lamp in the centre of the ceiling, aided by the light from the street outside. The lamp had hung over the centre of the dining table, and, as I lay there, memories came flooding back – of all that had gone on under the lamp, and round the family table, when we still had the family at home, and Mary had been fit and well, caring and catering for us all. When the simplest of objects, such as a lamp fitting, can be so evocative, such total recall can seem more of a curse than a blessing in the small hours.

In the morning, on the radio, "Thought for the Day" was, strangely enough, given by a dietician, who peppered his talk liberally with analogies drawn from his specialty. In particular, referring to the way in which our food residues passed through us, he stressed the need for us to be able to shed our past, and not to allow it to interfere with our experience of – and, indeed, our joy in – the present. A little crude as a metaphor, but I knew what he was getting at, and it was a lesson that I needed to learn, and re-learn, just then. Again and again I go back to Harry Williams: "to find our freedom in the fulfilment of our vocation, and to find our vocation in the inescapable fate put upon us by necessity, and thus to find a self which extends infinitely beyond the range of that confined cabined self which we imagined was all we were...."

I had discussed Harry Williams with Tom, and he had reminded me that he had known him well at Cambridge. There was a sense in which I felt I knew him too – just from his writings.

By that time I had already recorded the whole of the chapter on 'Resurrection and Suffering' from *True Resurrection*, so that I could listen to it in the car, or whilst I was about my business in the house, but I now have one of these sophisticated micro-recorders, whose tape cassettes, hardly bigger than a couple of postage stamps, yet take an hour's recording down each side. I have whole books summarised on them, which can be taken anywhere – on buses, on trains, or even on a country walk. There must be those who share a bus seat with me, or pass by on a country lane, who become aware of the white lead travelling up from an inner pocket to the little earpiece, via which such concentrated wisdom is pouring into my brain! – and they may well feel sorry for the man with the white hair and the matching earpiece, apparently cut off from the rest of the world by his deafness....

Cut off just then, maybe, but by the grace of God not yet deaf to the wisdom of those who have trodden the way before me, and have written where I may read.

Chapter Twelve

At the weekend, three days after Tom's visit, my younger son Roger and his wife Wendy, and their two little girls, arrived from Bath for an overnight stay, and the visit, even more vividly than Tom's, pointed up the vast differences between Mary's response and mine to such occasions: Mary, as ever, able to confine herself to the present moment, the Eternal Now, which for me was always likely to be overshadowed by a threatening aftermath.

They were 24 seemingly endless hours. The laughter of little children at play (yes, laughter again, and children's laughter this time, arguably the laughter of God himself) and the excited chatter of several people all talking at once round what had become for the time being the family meal table again. How Mary and I enjoyed that brief resurrection into family life again, and how much I enjoyed having Roger and Wendy to talk to, after Mary and the children had gone to bed!

Wendy and I shared a deep concern regarding the nature and origins of suffering, and, in particular the possibility always, of there being a masochistic element in it. We had discussed Harry Williams on previous occasions, and were soon back with him again. As he puts it, we like to feel that "we suffer because we are guilty," going on to imply that that is the sort of naivete we end up with "when we try to exorcise the brutality of the hard facts by fabricating explanations." He goes on, "Let us therefore abandon comprehensive [explanations] of suffering ... in order to examine at first-hand our own experience."

Speaking of four sculptures by Michelangelo, in which the figures look unfinished, he says, "The figures are emerging from rough stone as though they were tearing themselves out of it with tremendous effort and pain." He continues,

> In allowing us to see the cost of their creation, Michelangelo has revealed the cost of our creation. Those four figures are us as we are being torn out of non-being into being by the hammer blows of our experience, and we are being created not in spite of but because of them. Yet no more than the rough stone do we know what we are being hit into – what form or pattern of beauty is being revealed by the marks of the chisel. Yet a time may come when we are able to feel that somehow the experience of the hammer and chisel was worth it, that the experience has not after all reduced us to a mess of meaningless bits and pieces but has provided us with a value and richness we should otherwise have lacked, so that our suffering is now seen to be woven into our joy as an essential part of it. (p.163)

Paul got it right, I think, when he said, "The whole of creation groaneth and travaileth in pain together until now." Or, as The New

English Bible has it, "Up to the present, we know the whole created universe groans in all its parts as if in the pangs of childbirth."

Perhaps pain and travail are in the very nature of things an inevitable part of all creation and creativity. Or could it even be the other way round – that the pain and the travail are redeemed when we allow them to act creatively upon us?

Wendy and I were late to bed that night.

The departure the next afternoon of Roger and his family turned out to be a nightmare as far as I was concerned. The lunch was late, and then, in the middle of it, they realised that they had only just enough time to get back to Bath to keep another appointment. Suddenly, they were gone, vanishing round the sharp bend in the road only 50 yards from the house. How I came to hate that bend! And I had hardly closed the door on the vanished car when Mary said she was going to have her rest. Within little more than five minutes we had gone from all the busyness and bustle of a family meal to an empty dining room. Well – not quite empty, for I was faced with the all-too-eloquent aftermath of the meal: empty and half-empty dishes, dishes bearing the tell-tale marks left by those whose company had meant so much; marks which – just because they were all that visually remained of those so suddenly departed – one could hardly bring oneself to wash away. It was a moment of desolation, in spite of the fact that, in general, things were going so well for us. It meant, of course, that I hadn't yet succeeded in breaking "the manacles which chain us to the past" – that there was still much work to be done there.

After the washing-up, and as something of a distraction, I dealt with some practicalities, stripping the beds and getting the washing machine going. And after that I sat quietly, trying to recollect myself before getting Mary up again.

How best to cope with such visits? There was certainly a part of me that wanted to keep everything unchanged and unchanging, even our family, and our relationships with them. I wanted the comings and goings to be just as they had always been. But the one just brought to an end so suddenly had been different, and those to come would be different again, inevitably. It was back to Mary's 'Eternal Now'. Somehow I had simply got to learn to relish and savour the joys of the present moment.

> Joy is no joy
> Which needs to state its terms,

and the joys of the present moment are the only real joys we have – joy doesn't belong to the past or the future, it is essentially a matter of the here and now. Otherwise, there is no joy at all.

I could delay getting Mary up no longer. And it had to be a case of "steady as we go", for there must be no possibility of her getting even a glimpse of the last hour or two's turmoil: the sight of the car disappearing round the corner with its precious load; the aftermath of the meal; the thought that Roger and his family were already halfway to Bath; and the thought of Bath itself, the visits we used to make, and the question of how long it might be before we were able to go again – if ever.

Peggy rang that evening. It was strange how often she seemed to ring just when I was in need of her womanly wisdom. Or was it? It is easy to dismiss such occurrences as mere coincidence or, at best, serendipity. On the other hand it is easy too – all too easy – to see God's hand at work when life is going well for us, and to do our best to ignore his apparent absence when things go badly wrong; scoring the hits, so to say, and ignoring the misses. But, let's face it, such singular moments will never yield up their secrets to statistical significance tests, and we are left with our hunches – and what's wrong with that? Scientists have hunches too, and quite often have nothing more than hunches to go on, and will risk a great deal of time, energy, money, and even their reputation on them.

Peggy and I spoke at length of the plunge my feelings had taken that afternoon. She did not agree that it was a rather reprehensible bout of useless nostalgia or depression, or whatever. She thought it was much more likely to have been a flash flood of pure emotion, which had been dammed up for three months, with no normal outlet. There seemed to be some truth in that. She pointed out, too, that the kind of life I had been living was bound to take its toll: to the hospital, home again, 25 miles to work and back, shopping, DIY jobs at home, and back to the hospital at night; to say nothing of the fever state of emotion which had prevailed, throughout.

She was right, of course. At such times we seem to have a reserve energy tank, physical, mental, spiritual, which we draw on automatically, to tide us over, to see us through; but sooner or later there is a built-in warning that comes up on our mental control panel to tell us that even the reserve tank is getting low.

Peggy's phone call, so timely that it was difficult to regard it as accidental, made me aware again of the dashboard: of the light – if not a red one then at least an orange one – that was flashing there.

It took another eleven years, and Mary's death, to make me pay proper and due regard to it.

Chapter Thirteen

Autumn had thoroughly established itself by now, and we were well on into the 'second mile' of Mary's convalescence. We had been there before – in 1968 – and the combination was all too familiar. But (to use a vulgar but popular saying) how prone we are to shift the goal posts! Less than a month before, and with Mary coming home again in a matter of days, we were in our Seventh Heaven. And now, just three or four weeks on, the dead weight of the difficulties of the daily round was already beginning to tell. That seemingly ultimate goal of having Mary home, with all its looming joys, had been all but forgotten, and the days were increasingly a matter of overcoming some new crop of difficulties, with the crossbar already lowered to the modest height of merely getting through the day, and Mary safely in bed again, at the end of it.

The difficulties were not necessarily chronic ones, they would spring at us unexpectedly out of the undergrowth of the day, an amalgamation of smaller ones suddenly threatening to overwhelm us.

I remember, for example, one afternoon when I went to get Mary up after her rest. As so often happened when she first woke she was both more euphoric and (probably consequently) less able to follow what I was trying to get her to do; and a little less good, too, at standing, balancing, or whatever. A full half dozen times the poor soul swung round and flopped down onto the bed again as we tried to move off, and I completely lost my patience.

I found myself saying, "Do concentrate! Do help! My wrists are so stiff!" And I had to walk right away then for a few seconds to collect myself, and to stop getting really angry. I was appalled. I had to accept, of course, that I was only human, as they say, and that I was very tired. But the fact remained that for the first time I had allowed the difficulties to show through, and for the first time reacted to Mary as though she was fully capable and responsible, and was simply being awkward. It was, however, only the first of what were to be an increasing number of such occasions, staking out all too regularly that 'second mile', as it stretched out seemingly endlessly through the autumn and into the depths of winter.

I did my best to make it up to Mary, even trying to see a funny side of it with her, going back over it as though we had been doing a clowning act, in which I had stood her upright, and she had fallen over deliberately every time my back was turned! We had a wry laugh about it in the end, and she said, with her characteristically gentle good humour, "Not to worry! – you're forgiven."

Yet there was heart-searching again that evening as I was getting the meal, and heartache too, at the thought of all that had befallen us;

and I had to remind myself all over again of what my 'guru' Harry Williams had had to say about the need to allow the pain to be suffered to the full, because it is not simply the pain of our links with the past being broken, but the pain of being opened up forcibly to the future: the pain not only of dying, but of being born.

And I was reminded yet again when I put Mary to bed of the tenterhooks on which we were living, when she said she felt very tired. Any such remark and my heart would sink, fearing as ever that it heralded something much worse: it had been the same in the afternoon when we had had the trouble over getting her to stand, and she had said she couldn't feel very much in her ankle.

It certainly hadn't been an easy day. The aftermath of Roger and Wendy's visit still lingered on, raising the ghosts of a past existence which could never be recaptured. And the afternoon had been marred by my loss of patience. My heart had sunk, too, when Mary had asked to go to bed early yet again. There was no doubt about the loneliness then, with her asleep in another room, and most of the evening still to come. How different it had been when she was her old self, and we had had the whole evening to ourselves, together... I wondered for how long these early bedtimes would go on and, indeed, just how good they were for Mary, bearing in mind that she went to bed for a couple of hours in the afternoon, and didn't get up in the mornings anything like as early as she used to in the hospital. In fact, I had a little chat with her about it – and the need for her to have adequate time up and about, and to get a reasonable amount of exercise. But there it was: it was all to do with that 'second mile', wasn't it?

The evenings spent on my own became a time of stocktaking. For the first time I became aware of the need to give myself 'time off', though I was loathe to admit it. I thought of the tremendous relaxation it would be just to read a straightforward adventure yarn, like a Hammond Innes – yet I couldn't bring myself to do even that. Instead, I would do a bit more work on the paper I was writing; and one evening, as I worked, I became conscious for the first time of one of the more subtle problems with which we were having to deal during that 'second mile' of our journey.

I had been to the brink of death with Mary, and camped out there with her for days and weeks; and to come back to mundane things, such as writing a scientific paper, was an incredible kind of transition to have to make. One is returning almost literally from another world, and there is a need for kindness and sympathy (yes, even towards oneself) in the difficulties there are bound to be in making the return journey. It behove one not to attempt to sweep the difficulties under the carpet either: somehow one had to hold together in one's mind and spirit both the literally *awe*-ful time we had been through and the life of common day to which we had now to return.

After Roger and Wendy's visit I had been particularly conscious of the different levels at which our lives are lived. Perhaps the very existence of different levels was some kind of distortion of thought and feeling brought to light by the terrible times we had been through? If so, did the aberration belong to the past rather than to the present, then? Perhaps I had allowed myself to become far too preoccupied with the mundane, so that I just had not been ready and prepared for the crisis which can arise without warning in any of our lives – the ultimate crisis rooted in our very mortality:

> Early morning
> Gives no warning
> Of a sunset
> Less than eternity away:
> No need to plan the day.
>
> Mid-morning
> Is refreshment time –
> Let's take a breather
> From our play
> (The sunshine has surely come to stay!).
>
> High noon,
> And native powers
> Intoxicate
> With the sense
> That the choice is ours:
> There is nothing we could not do
> If we wanted to –
> But we don't.

I was back with the sentiments of the poem I wrote on my way to my sister's funeral nine years earlier. The crisis, of course, may not be distant, or cosmic, it may be 'just round the corner' – a street accident, or a diagnosis of cancer following some seemingly unimportant symptom. I could see the need to bring together, and to hold together, the (literally) deadly serious, and the (seemingly) trivial things of life. But how? Merely to contemplate such mundane activities as playing a round of golf ("They downed their beers, and swallowed their fears, that life might not be always a game") or even looking at some light-hearted offering on the 'box' would immediately sharpen all over again my perceptions and recollections of the crisis Mary and I had just lived through.

There was another side to it too. I realised that the crisis had brought with it not only some of the most terrible moments in our lives, but also experiences so profound that they made 'ordinary' life indeed seem trivial: but how to blend these two extremes into a unity again?

As autumn slowly and inexorably turned to winter, life for Mary and me gradually took on a sort of transient equilibrium. Days turned into weeks, weeks into months, and though progress was less spectacular from day to day, it was still discernible and significant. But, with hindsight, there was already a hint of a more chronic and insidious kind of equilibrium which later on, alas, came largely to characterise our life together.

In my tape diary at the time, there was an item which should have warned of the danger:

I am still finding the transition back to ordinary life very difficult, after all that we have been through. The problem lies in the dichotomy which I still feel to exist on the one hand between life lived on the heights, so to say, with the heightened consciousness which has gone with it these last four months, and on the other hand life lived at the mundane, 'everyday' level, which in my present state of mind, continues to seem so trivial.

The entry went on:

Should we, in fact, attempt to live on the heights all the time, so that nothing ever again appears trivial, and everything is always seen against the backdrop of eternity. Or is the nature of the human condition such that for the bulk of our time we need to have the eternal mediated by the mundane and 'the everyday'? Have we been living on heights which we cannot expect to occupy permanently, and from which we needs must descend again? I wonder?

It seems now that I should have gone on wondering: we had been through so much, and suffered so much to gain the heights; and as we left behind the acute stages of Mary's illness it was too easy, all too easy, to allow our daily lives to sink back once more into the mediocrity of common day.

The tape diary ended in late October, just as autumn turned to winter. I feel, however, that this was not the sole reason. There is evidence in a letter I had from Peggy at that time that the shades of the prison house were beginning to close on me again, that the dead weight of the daily routine, unalleviated any longer by any spectacular changes in Mary from day to day, was taking its toll, and I was beginning to murmur against my fate. With great subtlety she quoted those lines of Harry Williams back at me, which only a few weeks earlier I had quoted to her:

To find our freedom in the fulfilment of our vocation, and to find our vocation in the inescapable fate put upon us by necessity, and thus to find a self which extends infinitely in the literal sense (for it finds its identity in the Eternal Word) beyond the range of that confined cabined self which we imagined was all we were – that, in summary, is the experience of suffering and resurrection.

(*True Resurrection*, p.163)

It was a timely reminder, but much harder to take than it had been when I had quoted it to Peggy in the first flush of Mary's spectacular progress in Willow Ward. It was enough to put me back on the rails again (how often Peggy did that in those days!), but not enough to remove altogether the danger of that positive sense of vocation turning into a mere passive acceptance of the inescapable fate put upon us by necessity. And, in the years that followed, tragically and (dare I say it?) almost inevitably, that danger became the main threat to the quality of our daily life together, as we settled, so gradually, into that state of "chronic and insidious equilibrium."

Chapter Fourteen

On that bleak September Sunday afternoon, in the aftermath of the catastrophically sudden departure of Roger and his family back to Bath, I had wondered when, and whether Mary and I would together ever see Bath again: at the time such a journey seemed like a space odyssey merely to contemplate. Yet, as Christmas drew near, there seemed to be a desperate need for us to break out of the cribbing space of our own little house, which seemed to be shrinking by the day, and to know once more the liberating experience of new places and spaces, or the benediction of visiting old and familiar ones again.

I talked to our doctor about it. Was it mad, or at best plain foolhardy, even to contemplate the journey to Bath? (Roger and Wendy had already invited us for Christmas.) Greatly encouraged by the progress Mary had made, I think he was determined that we should not mark time – that we should reap such benefits as we could from that 'semi-heroic' action that he and the consultant had determined upon, way back in July.

"I should go," he said, adding something to the effect that I couldn't keep Mary wrapped up in cotton wool indefinitely, that there would always be a measure of risk involved in whatever we did (or didn't) do, and what better cause to take a risk for than Christmas with the family?

It is sad to think that nothing comes back to me of the festivities of that Christmas: just two things, very practical matters both of them, come to mind. The one was that I failed to pack the 'Stand-Easy', a vital bit of equipment which we were hard-pressed to do without, and the other was one of those photographic snapshot-style memories – of Roger walking into our bedroom one morning near the end of our stay, and without any preamble whatever asking, "Why don't you move to Bath?" There were some town houses about to go up, he added, virtually on their doorstep, too – so, 'What about it?'

It took hardly a second to decide, and in little over six months we had taken up residence in Bath.

Back home again after Christmas, the mere prospect of the move, with its promise of family support near at hand as and when we needed it, gave a new aura to life. It is said that moving house and home is a trauma second only to bereavement. That might be true in the aftermath, and even in the prospect, where the move is involuntary, forced upon one by untoward circumstances, and at a time not of one's own choosing. But, for Mary and me, at that time, it promised a real alleviation of our circumstances, and whole new vistas to life.

It is true that we would be leaving the house which had been our home for almost 30 years, the house where practically the whole of our family life had been spent, and from which the family had been launched. But all that was already ten years back – years overlaid by Mary's troubles, each of them a mini-lifetime, with the years of the family that had gone before already receding into the blue haze of time's far distance, and threatening to disappear over its horizon. The time when we gathered round the family table (under that central light which I had contemplated in the small hours), and Mary was her old self, and fit and well, seems now to belong to another incarnation; but already, in 1977, such associations as remained for me of the family house and home were negative rather than positive ones, and I, certainly, was not troubled by the thought of leaving it behind.

I don't know about Mary. She was certainly looking forward to living in Bath, but what kind of a wrench with the past it was for her was quite impossible to tell. Indeed, that was part of my own private and perpetual heartache (did I almost say 'hell'?) – not to know what her deepest feelings were about anything, any longer. It's terrible put as baldly as that, but that is how things were for us after that second stroke. There were those who said that in some ways it could be regarded as fortunate – that Mary was 'protected' from the full impact of events, particularly the more traumatic ones. But would that have been her choice? I am sure it wouldn't. Maybe she was not 'protected' in that way at all: maybe she just wasn't able any longer to express what she thought about events, and about what they were doing to her? But what comfort could that be? The harsh truth was that momentous decisions – such as whether or not to move house – could no longer be made jointly: it lay with me to decide what the effect on Mary, and on her quality of life, would be. It was an agonising responsibility.

Nevertheless, such problems went unacknowledged between us and as far as the move was concerned, had seemingly little effect on the pleasurable anticipation of being nearer to at least some of the family again. Moreover, we had no difficulty in selling the house, and soon arrangements were complete for the purchase of one of the town houses (it was only a foot high at the time!) which would be barely a hundred yards from Roger and Wendy.

Just six months later, on June 30th, we moved.

Logistically, moving house is the largest operation any of us are likely to be involved in, in ordinary life, and there is plenty of scope for something to go awry; and our move was no exception.

For instance, it would hardly seem possible for the van to have arrived within thirty or so yards of the house, and yet take another twenty minutes actually to reach it.

The problem was that the house was in 'Holloway', but the builders had always referred to the whole development as 'Carlton Gardens';

so, in my innocence, I had told the removal firm that the address was 'Holloway, Carlton Gardens'. What I didn't know was that there was an actual road called 'Carlton Gardens', and that, moreover, it was a cul-de-sac that ended in a turning place just thirty yards from our new house, at the top of a grassy embankment, with only a footpath connecting the two.

Dancing from one foot to the other with impatience in the empty house, and with the van already an hour late, I happened to look out of the window just in time to see it arrive at the turning place and grind to what must have been a very frustrated halt. I rushed up the embankment and intercepted them before they could make their getaway, to be told by the driver, with some emphasis, not to say anger, that they had arrived in the vicinity of 'Carlton Gardens' as he put it "the best part of an hour ago", to be told finally by a passer-by that 'Holloway' was "just at the end of the road"...

It was getting on for a couple of miles round the city to get to us and, when they eventually arrived, the prevailing mood was not exactly one of cooperation. How better to make up time than to bring the furniture in at the double, and do their best to ignore any remarks by me from the touch-line, as to where it should go? It was a 'town house', and apart from a tiny vestibule three feet square, one walked straight into the sitting-room. They did take the main bedroom furniture upstairs, but almost everything else ended up in that sitting-room, which looked like an overcrowded furniture storeroom by the time they had finished. As a parting shot, surveying their handiwork with some satisfaction, one of the men said, "Looks as though you could have done with a bigger house, guv," – and they were gone.

Fortunately, we had arranged to stay with Roger and Wendy for a few days, so I was able to shut the door on it all for a little while. But it was only the beginning of our troubles. Once we started trying to live in the house, we ran into a whole crop of further snags, most of them 'teething problems', to do with the fact that it was a brand-new house.

Thus the washing machine, quite indispensable, was as yet not plumbed in, but was fitted with a hook-on waste pipe, which I had hitched over the kitchen sink; and one morning, a day or two after we had moved in, I had left it with a load of clothes to wash whilst I went upstairs to get Mary up. Yes – that's it! The waste pipe unhitched itself from the sink, and discharged what I estimated to be about 25 gallons of water onto the kitchen floor. Because the house was 'open-plan', the sitting room was just round the corner from the kitchen area, and by the time I arrived on the scene again a fair proportion of the 25 gallons had been taken up by the new sitting room carpet: several square yards of it were squelching with water. It was a thick, all-wool carpet, and I had visions of it shrinking inches away from the wall in no time at all.

I panicked, and got out the vacuum cleaner (and I a scientist!). After removing a significant amount of the water from the carpet there was a sheet of blue flame from the cleaner, and the motor caught fire.

The next afternoon, and the house seemed to have been taken over by a whole group of tradesmen. There was a plumber in the kitchen plumbing in the washing machine, an Electrolux engineer fitting a new motor to the vacuum cleaner, two television engineers, one by the set, and the other in the loft, trying (unsuccessfully) to position an aerial for optimum results; and bringing up the rear, an electrician in the lounge endeavouring to find out why the central heating was switching itself on and off every half minute or so, of its own accord.

The washing machine duly got plumbed in, and the new motor fitted to the cleaner; the two television engineers departed crestfallen when I told them the picture was no better than it had been before, and waived their charges, whilst the electrician triumphed when he discovered that a carpenter had neatly driven a nail between two wires leading to the thermostat. A good time was had by all, and Mary and I were finally left in peace, glad to be on our own once more. We had had a surfeit of company for one afternoon.

Despite all this, Mary, in her inimitable way, had pronounced her own verdict on the move. It was after I had put her to bed the very first night we slept in our new home. Snuggling back into the pillows, she said, quietly but solemnly, "This house shall be called 'Content'". Just one word, but it left me speechless.

One can have an oasis in time as well as space, I suppose, and like that, Mary's oasis of content lasted less than three months.

As I walked into the bedroom with her breakfast one morning in September, she was in a torpid state, her features contorting rapidly in the horrifying way with which I was all too familiar, and in a matter of minutes she was deeply unconscious.

Our new doctor came, clutching her notes, and immediately ordered an ambulance. As they carried Mary out, he made an opportunity to speak to me on the side.

"You know," he said, soberly, "your wife is, I think, every bit as ill as she was last year." He had no reason to think otherwise, and I had no reason to hope otherwise, as I climbed into the ambulance with Mary. The scenario was indeed a horrendously familiar one.

At the hospital she was rushed into a ward where there seemed to be an emergency team ready and waiting for her, and she soon disappeared behind the curtains, with at least half a dozen people round her bed. The place was bustling and bristling with activity, and I took heart, feeling somehow that Mary had fallen into good hands. I rang Roger, and a little later he joined me on the bench outside the ward. Yet another vigil had begun.

We were offered the statutory 'cup that cheers', but it would have had to have been a very special one to cheer me just then. I was discovering that my feelings and emotions, which seemed to have recovered their resilience after the move to Bath, were actually almost as played out as they had ever been. It was as though that deeper level of being which had been so totally engaged in the battle for Mary in 1977 had fallen asleep exhausted; and that, as I sat there with Roger, someone was shaking me violently, and saying, "Come on! Wake up! It's all happening again." Was that really what they were saying? And for a third time?

About noon, the ward sister suddenly materialised in front of us. I took a firm grip on reality then, for the first time that morning, and steeled myself for the worst.

She said, "You can come and see your wife now," adding then, with a twinkle in her eye, "She's a fraud, you know!" It wasn't the first time that Mary's powers of survival had educed such a response.

"She's a survivor!" I declared, as Roger and I swept through the doors into the ward, to catch a first glimpse of Mary.

Strange, isn't it? – that the drama of the hospital ward goes on behind closed curtains, and it is only when it is all over that the curtains are actually drawn apart. There was Mary, comfortably propped up against her pillows, smiling ("Fooled you again, didn't I"), all the contortion of her features gone, and looking as though nothing had happened – nothing, that is, except that she had woken up in a hospital bed, instead of her own, where she had pronounced that all was pure 'content', just weeks before.

She stayed in hospital about a fortnight, mainly so that they could thoroughly reassess her drug regimen. She was also taken to Bristol for a brain scan, which showed that the trouble had been on the left side again. However, it had had only relatively minor effects on her mobility and her speech. We had been let off so lightly, compared with the previous year, but the incident inevitably undermined the growing sense of security we had begun to feel as a result of the move to Bath.

In January, 1979, Mary had yet another stroke, a very minor one this time, which had little or no effect on her, except on her confidence to climb the stairs – and we were marooned in the sitting-room for a fortnight.

Although we had been in the house only six months, this incident made me aware of a serious snag which the open-plan layout held for us in the longer term. Apart from the alcove comprising the kitchen area, the whole of the ground floor was a single, open dining-cum-sitting space. There was no way in which we could have set aside part of it as a bedroom. The house was an end one of a terrace of four, and, in the previous autumn we had already had built on to the end wall a downstairs loo and utility room, but to add a bedroom as well would have been quite impossible. Despite the fact that our bedroom had been downstairs in our old house, numerous dress rehearsals up and down the stairs there had convinced us that we would be able to manage. But we hadn't reckoned on Mary taking just one step down one day, and then, losing her nerve, sitting down on the top step, unable to move either up or down.

I got Helen, one of our new neighbours, to help us down to the bottom, only to find that Mary didn't want to have anything more to do with the stairs, at any rate for the time being.

Even prior to this little contretemps, we had become aware of other problems. Holloway was a steep hill, and there was no little 'rounder' that we could take for Mary's 'constitutional', as there had been in the case of our old home. Day after day, all we could do was to walk up the road fifty yards or so (which was as much as Mary could manage of the hill) and back again. It got very boring for both of us, and Mary began to show less and less inclination to take her walk each day.

That wasn't the only thing that turned out to be different from what we had imagined. Although the house was indeed only a hundred yards ('as the crow flies') from Roger and Wendy's, there was no direct road, not even a direct footpath. It was in fact the better part of a mile to them by car, and, as if that wasn't bad enough, the entrance to their little private road, between two stone walls, with a sharp turn immediately beyond, I found almost impossible to negotiate; and it wasn't long before I had scraped the side of the car on one of the walls. It was my turn to lose my nerve then; and after that, whenever we visited, Roger had to fetch us and take us home again – not exactly what we had envisaged before the move.

We began to realise that, being so near and yet so far from them, we might as well be a mile or so in some other direction altogether, and living in a bungalow. The trouble was that whilst there were quite a lot of bungalows in Bath, the very raison d'être of most of them was vitiated by the fact that they had a flight of steps up to them, or down to them, as the case may be.

But in a gentle sort of way, from then on, the hunt was on for a bungalow on a level site.

It took us nearly four years to find one.

In the meantime, life was by no means one long succession of newly unearthed snags. We began to realise the advantages of living in the West Country, within little more than an hour's journey by road (Mary's limit) from such places as the Wye Valley and Exmoor, and for six years, beginning in 1980, we ventured on annual holidays again. I say "ventured" advisedly, because we both needed to screw up our courage to leave behind the relative security of our home base, and take up residence, with all our bits and pieces, among a group of strangers, as hotel guests. But, apart from some almost inevitable contretemps, mostly it worked out well enough.

Nonetheless, in the Spring of 1980 I took myself off to the doctor's on my own behalf. I was feeling somewhat played out, and rather under the weather.

The doctor was reassuring, but followed up his verdict with a suggestion which I think I must have momentarily misunderstood completely, as raising again the whole question of Mary's 'institutionalisation' (the word is as ugly as it is long, and was as unacceptable as ever, to me). I heard him saying something to the effect that he could "get Mary into a home" if I wanted him to.

All I can remember then was of rounding on him fiercely, and saying, "Oh, no you don't – she's mine."

A moment later, and I think we both felt more than a little embarrassed, as he went on to explain that he had meant only for a week or two, to give me a break. I calmed down after that, and said I would think about it. It was the first time anyone had ever suggested such a thing, and for some subtle reason or other I was suspicious of the whole idea. It seemed innocuous enough, and still does in principle, but as I came to accept the argument that I needed regular breaks from the daily round of caring, all sorts of ramifications and conflicts grew out of its implementation, for both of us.

It was argued on my behalf (by others, and genuinely enough, I may say) that, apart from a few hours on a regular basis each week, I should also have an annual break of a week or two. Thus it came about, in the autumn of 1980, that a place was found for Mary in a pleasant 'Holiday Home for the Disabled', whilst I went off with Peggy's husband Clifford to Malawi for three weeks, to stay with Peggy's doctor daughter.

It was a wonderful time for me, but I was not at all convinced that it had been of unalloyed benefit to Mary. The trouble was the old and agonising one – that I just couldn't be sure that I had got through to her, as I tried to set out the reasons why such arrangements were coming to be considered necessary. In consequence, the arrangements came to feel increasingly unilateral, and almost imposed on Mary. Worse still, as they became part of the fabric of our lives, and I had to agree to Mary "going into hospital" when there wasn't a place for her in the Holiday Home, it turned out on more than one occasion that 'hospital' meant a geriatric ward of the kind that had given me nightmares when Mary was first admitted to Dr W's Unit. In no way could I purchase a respite from the daily round at such a price for Mary; and it was only by regularising the arrangements with the Holiday Home that I could contemplate continuing to take such breaks.

Even so, as the years went by, and Mary's difficulties gradually increased, she became more reluctant to agree to going to the Home at all, even for a few hours each week, let alone for a week or two, each summer.

Once again, in retrospect, I am conscious of the terrible and seemingly inexorable erosion of the quality of life and relationships that was going on in so many little ways, under the sheer dead weight of the daily round. It was, indeed, like "a bereavement in slow motion."

During the remaining eight years of Mary's life, there were no further major crises – that is, until the final one; and, looking back it seems now that we had become moulded by crisis, our lives geared to it, like those who, having already been through so many battles in a war, subconsciously hold themselves permanently in readiness for the next one to break out.

That was certainly true of me, but what of Mary and her capacity to live in 'The Eternal Now'? Had that changed, too? Had her capacity to live the life of 'pure spirit', in which the over-arching future was properly discounted, been finally eroded by that daily sense of threat of still further battles to come? I just do not know, and there, it must be said, lay the agony of it.

What I do know is that, over those remaining months and years, her zest for many of the ordinary activities of life was certainly being eroded – like going out for a ride in the car, for instance, or for that matter going anywhere at all, even for going on holiday. Increasingly, she wanted just to sit at home and read, and to receive visitors – she never lost her zest for that – until what turned out to be the last few weeks of her life.

Were we just holding our breath then, during those eight years, waiting for the next crisis to happen? Maybe – but when it came, it came by stealth, via the back door, neither of us for the time being recognising it for what it was.

There was one event during those last eight years which did change our daily life quite dramatically, particularly the mechanics of it – and that was the move to a bungalow, and a bungalow on a level site, too.

It was our friend Helen who spotted it in a house agent's window, as she was passing. Helen was one of that rare breed of people who actually enjoy moving – and second only to moving herself was the vicarious pleasure and satisfaction she got out of house hunting for other people. She was certainly responsible for giving Mary one of the last pleasurable changes in her life. After we had settled into the bungalow, how often Mary would say, as she traversed the few steps across the hall from the bedroom to the sitting-room, "I do like this little house!"

As ever and always though, the move, and almost everything connected with it, turned out to be far from straightforward. It was, in fact, one of those few occasions when I had to bare my teeth, so to say, on Mary's behalf. The fact was that the house agents had two offices, in different parts of the city, and they each sold the bungalow separately, to different people, one of whom was me. In other circumstances, and not being by nature an aggressive person, I would probably have bowed out politely. But not this time, and in the melée that followed I fought like a tiger on Mary's behalf, for I knew all too well what the bungalow would mean to her (and, let's admit it, to me too, in the sheer mechanics of daily living). Inevitably, it led to our being gazumped, something which I would normally have refused to be party to, but this was jungle warfare, and, "in the forests of the night", my eyes were certainly "burning bright", and the "fearful symmetry" of my argument of Mary's case must have given the house agents grounds for the sober reassessment of the less than satisfactory part they had played in the whole affair.

So, we moved house again in September 1982, four years after the move to Bath. My own particular contribution to the general mayhem was grossly to underestimate the time it would take to pack up on my own, so that Roger and Wendy and I were up till past 3 o'clock on the morning of the move, following a panic phone call to them at 10 o'clock at night. What bricks they were – and they both had to go to work the next day, too.

For the time being at any rate, the move was a shot in the arm for both of us, and provided a good deal of valuable occupational therapy for me – so much so that the usual autumn blues were kept at bay till near midwinter. Roger and I spent several weeks fitting out a whole new kitchen, which, at the time of the move had consisted of nothing more than a sink unit and a single wall cupboard. With my particular interest in cooking, it was wonderful to end up with a kitchen that had been planned exactly to my requirements.

The blues set in early in December, when we had arranged for a plumber to come. There was major work to be done, but he had a considerable reputation for high standards of workmanship, so that December had been the earliest we could book him. He had to instal a full gas central heating system and a new bathroom suite. Apart from the aesthetic aspects, the bath needed to be as low as it was possible to get it, if I was to continue to be able to bath Mary.

The trouble was that all this was to take about a fortnight, during which time the house would be quite impossible for Mary to live in. So, it was arranged for her to go into hospital for that period, and in the event it turned out to be the worst of all possible worlds: a traditional geriatric ward, and in a small town twenty miles out of Bath. It was bad enough living rough for a fortnight in a cold house littered with the constituent parts of our central heating system-to-be, together with all the plumber's tools of the trade; but to visit Mary each day, seemingly banished from Bath to a grossly overcrowded and (ironically enough) grossly overheated hospital ward, packed with patients with whom she could make hardly any meaningful conversation... It became yet another of those images, plastering the walls of that mental photographic gallery of mine, as stark and as painful now as it was when it was etched in, nine years ago.

But it must be acknowledged that in the last analysis it was all in a good cause, and, like Christmas '77, when Roger had first mooted the move to Bath, Christmas '82 was again something of a milestone – our first in our new, all-on-one-level home, and a warm and cosy one too.

Chapter Fifteen

Despite the new bath, with its edge a mere 17 inches from the floor, bath-times became increasingly difficult for us. We had long since used a seat across the bath, and the height of the new bath made it exactly level with the box seat beside it. The idea was simply to slide Mary from one seat across and onto the other, having first lifted her feet over the edge of the bath.

The trouble was that she weighed more than I did, and what looked easy on paper turned out to be not nearly so easy in practice. So, to overcome the difficulties, and to avoid bath-times becoming hassle-times as well, we finally arranged for a nursing assistant to come once a week to bath her.

It was a good move. Indeed, what had been rapidly becoming a fraught occasion was converted overnight into a relaxed and happy one for Mary. After all, it meant another regular visitor each week; and the sound of Mary's voice emanating from the bathroom, as she chattered away to the nurse about her work and her family, is still a vivid and treasured memory.

Thursday morning was bathtime, and Mary would stay in bed after breakfast until the nurse came. Then, in dressing gown and slippers, she would cross the hall with the nurse, on the way to the bathroom. It was a moment of respite for me, when I could feel that for a little while Mary was safe in someone else's hands.

I was sitting at the dining table, enjoying a leisurely cup of tea, the door into the hall wide open. I looked up suddenly then, my eye movement like that of a camera shutter, capturing yet one more of those fleeting mental images – only this time it was recorded complete with its verbal caption:

> I saw you
> On the nurse's arm,
> Head tilted forward,
> Shoulders bent;
> Right foot sideways,
> Hobbling,
> And my heart
> Was rent.

It was 1987, and with the benefit of yet more hindsight, it is so clear to me now that spiritually I was beginning to live from hand to mouth, and Mary's courage, though as unflinching as ever, was becoming steadily more stoical, by the day.

Neither of us had either the will or the heart to go on holiday that year, and we had the first (and the last, as it turned out) of what I called our 'nominated' holidays. The idea was to designate ten days or so as holiday time, when we would go out as many times as possible for rides in the car, and have as many meals out as we felt like. But, when it came to it, neither of us could muster much enthusiasm for the arrangement. It is obvious, now, that by then we were each trying to flog a very tired horse. But it wasn't obvious then.

Instead, for me, it presented itself as a sort of accidie, a sickness of the spirit, the onset of which filled me with little short of horror:

Not to get used
To the sound of your foot
Dragging reluctantly
Across the floor
Behind your walking frame,
Which you manoeuvre
Like an unwilling mule
You are desperately trying
To tame;

> Not to get used
> To the sight of your face,
> Frustration-fraught,
> As you strive for the word
> That is pikestaff-plain
> To your inner eye –
> But you struggle to say
> In vain;

Not to get used
To the clutch of your hand
On my arm
As we dare the two steps
To the garden below –
A journey whose hazards
You, only, can know;

> Not to get used
> To the thought
> That once was a time
> When foot followed foot
> In so graceful
> A walk,
> And word followed word
> In a torrent
> Of talk,
> And arm tucked in arm
> Just for love
> Not support;

God!
Not to get used
To these things,
I say –
Not to get used to them, God,
I pray...

... words wrung out of me in July, when I was all too conscious that 1987 was the tenth anniversary of Mary's entering Willow Ward. Indeed, they were entitled, "Ten Years On."

Earlier, I have said that I was unaware of what had prompted me, in August 1987, to listen for the first time in those ten years to the tape diary of the Willow Ward days. But I know now that it was just that sense of anniversary – and the awareness that there was no longer another Willow Ward beckoning – that sent me back to the tapes, in the hope of revitalising a flagging spirit, as I listened to the account of those few brief, miraculous weeks.

September, October and November were spent bent over my desk in the corner of the sitting-room transcribing, longhand, the six hours of tapes. I had no word processor then, or even a typewriter, and ended up with hundreds of pages of almost illegible manuscript which had to be copied out a second time in as fair a hand as I could manage, before I dare pass it on to a typist. Even so, the whole thing had to be typed out twice before we finally got it right (the typist failing to follow the basic rule of her calling as a copy-typist – she had her own unique spelling and ideas on punctuation!).

Consequently, it was January 1988 before I was able to present Mary with her copy of that first (and much more slender) version of *Your Sort of Courage*. I remember it feeling a bit like "This is Your Life" as I did so. Little did I know how near to being so it actually was; for in six months, Mary had died.

She read it through at a single sitting that same evening, and made just two comments, both so poignant in their different ways, but neither showing any sign of a new spirit or a new purpose stirring within her, as a result. I realise now that she was very near the end of her tether by then.

The first comment came part of the way through. She looked up with the strange and almost bizarre expression I had come to know so well. Ever since that first stroke in 1968 she had been deprived of the very mechanism of weeping – no tears, no sobbing, just that expression of hers – depicting all too plainly the agony of her deprivation.

She said, bleakly, "This makes me cry."

If she could have found the words, she would have said, "This makes me want to cry, but I can't." The pain of it was writ large in her features. Yet something told me that had she been able to weep just then, the tears would not have been of sorrow or sadness, but of pure emotion. And that was a great consolation.

The only other thing she said was at the very end, as she closed the book. It was typical of her, and so utterly self-disregarding. Nonetheless, it was a moment of sorrow and anticlimax for me, for I had been desperately hoping that the record of the Willow Ward days, shared for the first time between us, would stimulate many happy memories, and give us both new heart.

With obvious regret, but, I felt, more than a little tired in spirit, she said, quite simply, "I didn't know that you'd had to give up your golf."

And that was all.

"Looking back," said John, "it could have been basically that Mum's immune system was failing."

John, our older son, is an organic chemist, and in drug research. He was speaking just after Mary had died, in July 1988, and he was looking back over the first six months of that year, at a whole series of disparate and seemingly unrelated things that had been happening to her.

She had had two bouts of 'flu, one in the New Year, and another in the Spring. At the turn of the year, too, she had developed a small ulcer on her ankle, where the lower strap of her caliper had rubbed. Nothing like that had happened before, over the many years she had had to wear the caliper. The ulcer stolidly refused to heal. She had complained of a sore mouth, which gradually became peppered with tiny ulcers which came and went, sometimes seeming to respond to antibiotics, at other times seeming to be totally resistant. She had had an ingrowing toenail, too, which had repeatedly festered, which, combined with the ankle ulcer, made walking difficult and very painful at times. As if that weren't enough, she began to have 'waterworks' problems again, particularly during the night.

The trouble was that in the small hours this problem would often look to be mere obstinacy to me, or even mildly perverse behaviour on Mary's part, as though she no longer wanted to bother. We had a long-established routine for night-times, which involved my being out of bed for two or three minutes only, the intention being to forestall any likelihood of an accident with the bedclothes. But one of the most painful memories I have to live with now, belongs to the small hours just two nights before Mary went into hospital for the last time. I had had to change the bed twice, and after the second time I was very tired, and very cross, and I remember saying to Mary, "You know, you're lucky I haven't smacked you." It was not, of course, meant seriously – simply as an indication of how I felt.

It is true that when I climbed into bed for the final time at 4 o'clock I had simmered down, and as I stroked Mary's head to get her off to sleep (whilst frantically trying to stay awake myself long enough to achieve that end) I said to her gently, "Let's treat the whole thing as some sort of nightmare, shall we? – and go to sleep now." And off she went.

But when John came out with his comprehensive diagnosis, all the impatience and misguidedness of my view of events in the small hours came home to roost. Poor Mary – I had been talking about smacking her, albeit jokingly, for what had probably been a bladder infection.

It all seems so plain now as one looks back, but at the time it was by no means so. With hindsight, I might have responded so differently to those events of the first six months of 1988, and which turned out to be the last six months of Mary's life.

As it was, the bare bones of the situation were that Rosemary was scheduled to come from Germany in July, with her little boy, to spend their summer holiday with us, and somehow or another we needed to get Mary into better shape, so that she could enjoy their stay; and I needed the time to get ready for it.

Life was rapidly becoming more and more like a juggling act, but how to bring the juggling to an end tidily, with all the clubs in the air and me desperately, still, trying to keep them there? I had arranged for the community nursing sister to call on the morning of Tuesday, June 14th, to discuss our plight. It was the day preceding all our troubles in the small hours; and such, already, was my mental state that I forgot all about the arrangement with the nurse. John our friend, and Anglican priest, was due to come on his regular monthly visit, to bring communion to us; but, less than an hour before he was due, Mary suddenly said, without warning, preamble, or explanation, that she didn't want to take communion.

It is true that, the day before, she had unaccountably turned her hairdresser away, though she, too, had come by arrangement. I could just about accept that, though even that was out of character, for Mary normally looked forward to having her hair done. But communion was a very different matter. It meant so much to us, and though I eventually succeeded in persuading her to go through with it that Tuesday, the mere fact that she had questioned it was a heartbreak; and when I answered the ring at the door as the nurse arrived to keep the appointment that I had forgotten, my eyes were puffed with the tears that I had hastily wiped away.

Her first words were, "Oh, you are in a way, aren't you? Let's come in and try and sort something out."

And that, fatefully, was when it was arranged that Mary should go into hospital for a couple of weeks, to give me a chance to make ready for the holiday we were to spend with Rosemary and her little boy, and to give Mary the chance of having her festering big toe, her ulcerating ankle, and her sore mouth attended to, all under one roof.

She was to go in on the following Friday: it would be June 17th. Even then, before I could have had any inkling as to how events were to turn out, I saw it as a cruel twist of fate that it should be the very day of the 20th anniversary of Mary's first stroke.

But it was to be much more than a mere coincidence of dates.

That Friday morning the ambulance arrived punctually. The lady who came once a week to do some housework was with us, a fact which led to yet another of those mental images burnt indelibly, as if by a flash bulb, onto the retina of my mind's eye. They didn't use a stretcher – the two ambulance men carried Mary out on a sort of chair. And as they turned at the foot of the front-door step, Mary looked back at our friend and waved, as cheerful as ever, and called out, "See you again soon!" But five weeks on, our friend was placing on Mary's grave a lovely bouquet of flowers: and on it was inscribed, simply, "To a lovely lady."

As the ambulance doors closed on Mary, I jumped into the car then, and set off for the hospital. I wanted to be there when she arrived, so that she didn't feel alone.

Chapter Sixteen

The hospital was not far, little over a mile perhaps, and Mary had been there before, twice in fact – once so that I could go away, and the other time to get her on her feet again (literally and metaphorically) after a bad bout of 'flu and bronchitis in the winter of '81. So, there was just a touch of 'home from home' about it. We were both familiar with the place and, much more important, it was modern in both appearance and function – for the elderly it's true – but as an acute, short-stay Unit only, so that there was nothing of that 'hangover' from a Poor Law institution that had characterised at least two of the other units that she had stayed in.

Moreover, she wasn't acutely ill – anyway, not when she was admitted: she would be out again in a fortnight, wouldn't she? – and Rosemary and her little boy would be arriving shortly after that. We could put behind us those fraught days and nights we had just been through; there was so much to look forward to now.

There was certainly nothing depressing about the ward. On the second floor of a modern block, it was light and airy, and arranged in relatively cosy six-bed bays, all accessed from a spacious concourse, halfway along which was Sister's desk, where the nurse in charge sat, when writing or consulting patients' notes, or just sitting, if ever there was the time to do simply that.

Mary was put into a corner bed alongside a large window, at the remote end of one of the bays. This was in itself both a treat and a sort of privilege, for it meant that for once Mary was not an emergency case, placed under the nose of the nurse in charge, where a close eye could be kept on her. It was all part of the false sense of security, though, into which we were being lulled.

Nevertheless, Mary's hospitalisation just at that time, and the manner of it, bestowed on me one great blessing which nothing could take away, not even the fatal turn that events took later on – especially, indeed, not that.

Suddenly, I was free of all the hassle and worse, of caring for Mary physically, and was able, so to speak, to be truly separate from her – almost for the first time, it seemed. The all-embracing nature of the physical caring for so long had brought about a kind of fusion, and, indeed, of confusion, between our very states of being. And it was as though I had been released from the bondage that Mary's handicaps had day by day placed upon me, so that we could begin to relate to each other in a new freedom of spirit. The hours which we were to spend just being with each other, especially after that final, and eventually fatal stroke, were filled (dare I say it?) with a kind of glory not of this world.

Does that seem like spiritual arrogance? I hope not, for it is a simple, objective statement of how it was for both of us – that is, until Mary began to suffer the ravages of pneumonia, and even her calmness of spirit was overwhelmed then.

The evening before Mary was admitted was spent carefully constructing a list of what needed to be attended to: the infected toe nail, the ankle ulcer, the redesign of her caliper, to avoid a recurrence; a reassessment of her walking with, perhaps, the need for some physiotherapy; and, of course, her sore mouth – a mention too of 'waterworks'.

It looks a formidable list now, and one which, it seems, should have given rise to more concern than it did at the time. But over-arching all at that moment was that wonderful sense of release from the grinding routine of each day, coupled with the thought that none of the items on the list compared in seriousness with a stroke in which, subconsciously, I went in daily fear on Mary's behalf.

The list went over onto the second side of an A4 sheet, and whilst they were putting Mary to bed (a little incongruously, it seemed then, as I had only recently got her up) I hove to in front of the young doctor sitting at the desk, explained who I was, and handed him the sheet. He looked a little askance at it at first, his body language definitely suggesting that I had stepped out of line. However, I went on to explain to him that I might well not be present when they came to set up Mary's notes, and that with her very real difficulties with her memory, and some difficulties with her choice of words, they might have problems. His manner changed suddenly then and, carefully tucking my list into Mary's ready-and-waiting folder, he seemed to relax, prepared to allow his features to display the look of the harassed man he really was and happy to accept help from whatever quarter it came, as he thanked me.

That first night I left Mary at about 8 o'clock, tucked up in bed after her supper and settling in well, adaptive as ever to whatever was happening to her. What a blessing that always was – enabling me, as it did, to leave her without any qualms or fears on her behalf. In my 'days off' I had begun to paint, and I drove straight out into the country in search of a subject for the next day. The feeling of being released from the responsibility for Mary for the time being, and from "the tyranny of time" in its most mundane sense, was growing by the minute, and my state of mind as I drove off must have had something in common with that of a dog who, having been straining overlong at the leash, suddenly finds itself free.

I drove to Combe Hay in the gathering dusk, and sized up a little village scene which I had had my eyes on for some time, but decided against it; on to Freshford then, where it took no time at all to settle for the little bridge, with the Inn beyond it. The painting would take two afternoons, and I would go whilst Mary was having her lunch, followed by her 'statutory' afternoon rest. That would be something like three hours total each day, including getting there, and getting back again.

Saturday morning dawned bright and sunny, so much like that fateful morning in 1968 when Mary's saga had begun.

A post-breakfast visit found her settled in as well as I could have hoped. A little more euphoric than usual, perhaps, with her excited chatter about the nurses and ward staff, but that was all. She hadn't selected who was to be 'my nurse' yet, but a short list was already emerging. In such a place, a short list of 'ogres' was inevitable, too – isn't that how we all tend to cope, under stress? Anyway, it was one of the more endearing traits of Mary that her abiding interest in people was such that, given a change of circumstances which produced a whole new crop of faces, she would immediately home onto a new face, hardly conscious of whether the 'place' which had produced it was a hospital or a holiday hotel. She might have her favourite nurse, but it wouldn't be long before some of the nurses would have a favourite patient, too.

The ward was short-staffed, particularly, it seemed, at the weekends, when an admixture of part-time staff would appear, both nursing and ancillary, and there was certainly a dearth of doctors, except for emergencies of course. So that, even on that first Saturday morning, it became obvious that nothing very much was going to happen as far as Mary was concerned until Monday morning, when the consultant was due to make his round. Even then, of course, we weren't expecting anything dramatic, for wasn't it all something of a routine for Mary, and just a break for me?

The painting went well, and, in those almost halcyon days of Mary's first week in hospital, it produced a little episode in the middle of Sunday afternoon which was so much the product of my relatively carefree mood.

I was painting by a little footpath that led across a grassy meadow, and the fine weather had produced the usual crop of Sunday afternoon ramblers. I hate onlookers when I am painting, but the job was nearly finished, and had turned out well enough for me not to be bothered overmuch with hiding it from the passers-by. One group of these was a whole family, Mum, Dad, and two or three kids. Strangely, it was Dad who was curious, not the children this time. He hung behind, and began to express his appreciation, which I immediately brushed aside. I had just finished reading a book (it had taken me many weeks) called *Drawing from the Right Side of the Brain*, and it had really convinced me that, given the correct approach, anyone – yes, anyone – could draw and paint competently. I said as much to the man. I was already convinced that he was a visitor on holiday from somewhere within earshot of Bow Bells. "Don't give me that Guv! As far as I'm concerned, it's a bloody miracle."

Be that as it may, it was the first (and the last) miracle with which I have ever been credited. Would that I could have worked one for Mary....

The painting, as I had been hoping, was finished by the end of Sunday afternoon, and by the end of Monday it was mounted and framed and ready to take along the next day to show Mary, as a little 'offering'. Painting it had been a rare treat, free as I had been of the usual constraint on the time for which I could absent myself: I was still feeling very much like that dog at last let off its leash.

The feeling was not to last for long however, for when I arrived at the ward at 10 o'clock on the Monday morning, Mary's bed was empty, and she was nowhere to be found. An anxious enquiry on my part produced the information that she had been taken to the X-ray department. This was certainly somewhat alarming, until I found out that the X-rays were something in the nature of a routine. How long would she be? They didn't know – could be quite a long wait, they said. I asked where the X-ray department was then: at least I could sit with Mary, if she also was 'just waiting'.

It was quite a walk, and when I eventually got there it was to find Mary stuck in her wheelchair on her own, in a long, bleak corridor.

She was so grateful. "I'm so glad you've come. I've had the X-rays, but I didn't know when anybody was coming to take me back again."

"Don't worry, love – I'll sit with you till they do." I daren't intervene and take her back myself, but the incident had stirred all my old anxieties again – of Mary caught up willy-nilly in the machinery of a large hospital – and there being little I could do to make sure things went smoothly for her.

I didn't have to wait long for another instance to arise. It was the next day, Tuesday, when I arrived for my evening visit, complete with the Freshford painting to share with Mary. Supper was over, but once again there was no sign of her – that is, not until I heard her voice (I had a job to locate where it was coming from at first) calling plaintively, "Nurse, nurse, can you help me?"

Fortunately she repeated it, and I was able to locate her then. She was in one of the loos, wedged, as she had been years before at home, between the loo itself and the wall. She said she had been calling for two or three minutes, but couldn't make anyone hear. These memories – of Mary a hostage to fortune in a large understaffed, overworked hospital – are such painful ones still. She seemed so forlorn, so vulnerable.

I showed her the painting, hoping that it would bring her a breath of fresh air, there within the four walls of the hospital, and be a little reminder of the countryside we both loved so much. It is true that just for a few seconds she did respond with a touch of her old spirit. But it suddenly gave way to a bout of euphoria, and some confusion, which I did my best to 'sweep under the carpet' there and then: I just didn't want to know about it.

There was trouble right at the beginning of the next day too, concerning the ulcer on her ankle. The staff nurse in charge that morning seemed to want to put her stamp on events and had removed the highly specialised dressing, which the community nursing sister had kept on it for months, under the instruction of our GP. I discovered it was missing when the physiotherapist was putting Mary's caliper on, prior to trying out her walking. She was a kindly, middle-aged soul, and highly experienced, who had met up with Mary several years before in one of those other hospitals. She had recognised Mary immediately, no doubt in her time having been adopted as 'my physiotherapist' – an honorary title not likely to be forgotten after being bestowed with the full weight of Mary's enthusiasm and gratitude!

I went straight off to the nurse concerned, who was sitting wearing the garment of authority as obviously as one might a new coat, all too conscious of its stiffness and straightness, and the lack of any comfortable creases in it. I gave her the benefit of the doubt. "I'm afraid the dressing on my wife's ankle seems to have got left off this morning," I said, ingenuously.

"It's not been forgotten," she replied, already showing some evidence of defensive irritation at the mild criticism which she might have considered my statement implied. "We decided to leave it off."

"But it's had that on for months," I remonstrated, "and as I understand it, it is the only type of dressing likely to give the ulcer a chance to heal, even though it may take a long time."

Her expression became more defensive and yet at the same time more determined. Here was someone, I felt, whose actions were being dictated less by her professional judgement than by some inner need to prove something to herself.

"It's for us to make such decisions," she said, almost curtly, and with more than a hint of impatience at the ill-informedness of the layman.

Was I stepping out of line? – even being a little paranoic on Mary's behalf? Be that as it may: at least I was the patient's husband, and there was no-one else around who was going to fight her corner for her.

I went back and unburdened myself to our friend the physiotherapist.

She said simply, but significantly, "Leave it with me." The next morning (Thursday) the dressing was back on again. But I had reason, much more serious reason, to doubt the judgement and motivation of that particular nurse later still, in the closing days of Mary's life.

The physiotherapist seemed reasonably satisfied with Mary's walking, but was less happy with her caliper, and said she would arrange for a visit from the man who would be responsible for making her a new one, if she needed it. I don't know what one would call such a craftsman, but craftsman he was, and he must have been on the premises that very day, for he came in the afternoon, and sorted out the details of a caliper which would minimise the risk of rubbing, and consequently of another ulcer, when the present one had healed.

But the new caliper arrived in the ward after Mary had had that final stroke, and she never wore it.

Meanwhile, on the Wednesday and the Thursday afternoons, whilst Mary was resting, I did another painting, this time of the weir at Avoncliff. I planned to get it mounted and framed on the Friday morning (I knew a framer who would do it whilst I waited), ready to take to Mary on the Friday afternoon.

I remember having a lively and forward-looking conversation on the telephone with Peggy that morning which did, in fact, delay my arrival at the hospital by a quarter of an hour or so. In the normal way it would have been of no consequence: I might well have found myself waiting on a seat on the ward concourse whilst they finished getting Mary up. And anyway, she would enjoy seeing Avoncliff again in the afternoon, even though it would be in the form of one of my rather amateurish paintings. Take things leisurely for once, I told myself, there really was no need for any hurry.

But when I came,
As usual,
Soon after breakfast-time,
And sought you in the day-room
In your favourite chair and place,
I found you, yes, I found you,
Oh! yes, I found you there;
But no-one, but no-one
Had found you'd lost your speech.

My poor beloved
Mary dear,
They told me that the nurse
Who got you up that day was new –
Would not have known that you could speak
The day before.

God! the horror of it all –
Even to me you looked the same
As I came up to your chair,
But when I asked, 'How's you today?'
All you could do was sit and stare,
Gesticulate at me
And murmur,
Incoherently.

To think that all in ignorance
They'd got you up,
And dressed you;
Put you in your wheelchair too,
And pushed you to the sitting-room
To wait for me to come;
And all that time,
My poor dear love,
You'd failed to make them understand
That you had had yet one more stroke –
Oh, God!
The horror of it all.

That was part of *Retrospect*, written a few months after Mary died: the horror is with me still, and as great as ever, three years on.

I dashed back as fast as I dare along the concourse to the nurse in charge at the desk.

"My wife has had another stroke," I blurted out, staying as calm as I could.

"Are you sure?" she asked, incredulous.

But a sobering thought struck her then. She spoke slowly, working out its implications as she went along. "It was a new nurse that got her up, she only came onto the ward this morning. It would have been the first time she had seen your wife...." She stood then, suddenly. "I will come and see her."

There was no doubt, of course, and Mary was taken straight back and put to bed again, whilst they called for a doctor.

Again, it seemed, just when my back was turned, Mary had suffered yet one more calamity.

Chapter Seventeen

It was natural to be making immediate comparisons: June 17th 1968; June 21st 1977, and now June 24th 1988. To add to the dreadful familiarity of it all, even the day of the week fitted, for June 24th was also a Friday in 1977. What was it about that third week of the month of June?

But there were other more helpful and more hopeful comparisons. Mary had not lost consciousness this time: indeed, mentally, she seemed more lively than she would normally have been so early in the day, though frustration would probably be a better word than liveliness to describe her state. Even that was some comfort, compared with the awful passivity of a comatose condition. One was clutching at every straw that floated by. There seemed to be full movement of both her arms, too (there was no means of assessing her leg movement just then), and she was certainly making good use of them to express her frustration. Mary was a great communicator, and loss of the means to communicate would weigh far more heavily with her than any loss of mobility.

Altogether, the comparisons seemed reassuring, inviting the conclusion that things were not as bad as they had seemed to be, under the impact of the shock discovery. After all, she had been deeply unconscious in the autumn of 1978, and had survived virtually unscathed. What I was failing to do (influenced by Mary's fighting spirit, and her capacity to survive, so amply demonstrated in the past) was to make proper allowance for the fact that she was 20 years older than she had been in 1968, and 10 years older than in 1978. There was John's point too, that her immune system was probably failing. With the benefit of his hindsight, I might have realised that the real threat to her lay elsewhere, and not with the stroke at all.

Tragically, such hindsight might also have benefited the nurse who was so eager to use the authority vested in her.

It was Friday afternoon, and the weekend was upon us again, when there would be the usual preponderance of part-time nursing staff on the ward, combined with the dearth of doctors. This meant that it would be Monday before any serious work on Mary's rehabilitation began – a thought born of my anxiety and impatience on Mary's behalf, rather than any serious lacks in the actual running of the hospital, apart from those springing from a perennial shortage of funds.

Fortunately, and as some sort of compensation for the enforced lull in the ward's activities over the weekend, it would be the consultant's ward round again on Monday morning, which at any rate (I thought) would get Mary off to a good start, at the beginning of the week.

The main fact to have emerged was that apart from having lost her speech again she had also lost her 'swallow reflex', which meant that she could not take solid food, and could not swallow even fluids properly. Most of the time at the hospital that weekend was spent trying to trickle water into her, whilst at home I developed a method of cooking four little plastic pots of egg custard simultaneously, in the microwave. They were perfect – and were to comprise a major item among the various foods I was to try so desperately during the next week or two to get Mary to take.

By the beginning of the week I had largely taken over her fluid intake chart. The target was a minimum of about 500ml a day, but it was rarely if ever achieved, and I was never sure how much of what I trickled into the side of her mouth as she lay back on the pillows actually went down her throat. What satisfaction there was when I was rewarded with the sound (and sight) of a feeble gulp which meant that the latest teaspoonful had found its way to its destination!

This task of mine was virtually a self-appointed one, the ward sister, perpetually short-staffed, only too happy to accept the help of another pair of hands more than eager to take on such a time-consuming task as trying to spoon in at least a pint of fluid a day, teaspoonful by teaspoonful.

In desperation I resorted to other methods too, including a spray intended for scent but filled with water, which I would use whenever Mary's mouth dropped open. The spray held 10ml, and I conscientiously recorded on the fluid chart each time I needed to refill it. Mary's mouth, still ulcerated, used to get so dry and parched, and how gratefully she used to hold it open sometimes to receive the cooling spray. There was so little one could do for her.

So far as fluid intake was concerned, I was clearly losing the battle, and after a few days she was put on a dextrose drip.

By Tuesday, June 25th, four days after the stroke, she had begun to perk up somewhat. When I arrived after breakfast she came out with the first four words she had managed to produce since having the stroke. She no sooner set eyes on me than she said simply, but very firmly, "I wan' come home."

It is rare indeed that something happens which makes one both very happy and very sad at the same time – it was so wonderful to hear Mary speak again so soon, but so terribly distressing not to be able there and then to fulfil her wish.

I found myself saying to her, quietly, earnestly, as though making her a solemn vow (which I was, of course), "As soon as the nurses and the doctors have got you just well enough for you to be able to come home, and for me to be just able to look after you again – that very moment you shall come home again."

We were looking straight at each other as I spoke, and Mary's eyes lingered a little, looking deep into mine, as though she was drinking in what I had said, then savouring it. It was one of those occasions, all too rare for many years, when I was able to feel that I had got right through to her. She didn't attempt to say anything more just then, but I felt sure I had convinced her. In the event, things took a turn for the worse in a matter of days, and that little cheery call to our friend as she had left the house only ten days before, "See you again soon," was never to be realised. But I take comfort now from the thought that after that little exchange between us she knew that nothing would stand in the way of her return home except some quite insuperable nursing problem.

For the rest of that morning, Mary and I were both riding high in spirit – and in hope too, I believe. She loved travel and nature books, and for her birthday that year I had bought her a book called *Nature of Australia*, and I had taken it along, to turn the pages over with her, and to talk to her about the wonderful pictures of the flora and fauna and landscape with which it was teeming. In retrospect I see such brief times, of which there were several in the first week following the stroke, as part of the lull before the storm which was to follow; and it was to lull me into all sorts of false hopes and expectations for the course that Mary's illness would take. As we sat there, thumbing through the pages together, the atmosphere of a hospital ward fell away from us, and we could almost have been in deck chairs on a holiday beach, taking the sun.

In the middle of this John, our friend and priest, arrived, and hard on his heels came Elizabeth, another of John's parishioners, who had been visiting Mary for almost the whole time we had lived in Bath. She was a prime example of one of those who had started visiting Mary to alleviate her largely housebound state, but who had soon fallen under her spell.

Their arrival led to another of those mental images destined to stay with me for the rest of my life – of Mary holding court, so to say, with the three of us. I was so thrilled that she had formulated her first four words, and I was regaling the others with this fact, and recounting other little incidents and hopeful signs that had occurred. And, as I did so, Mary, full of spirit, teased me with jaunty 'good old me' gestures, tossing her head, and thumbing imaginary lapels. What spirit she showed that morning! She actually sat there, four days after having a stroke, entertaining us.

How feeble my spirit, by comparison. By lunchtime the thought of the long haul that lay ahead of us yet again was bearing down on me, grinding out of me the joy that I had experienced earlier, when I had joined Mary in her 'Eternal Now'; and soon I was watering the morning's brief heaven with my tears again. They were the old tired, tormented tears for the Mary of twenty years before, and for all that might have been.

For one brief hour I was to "Rage, rage, against the dying of the light," as I scrimmaged and scrabbled for words to express the dark anger that had erupted from my depths.

The words fizzled out though, the anger quickly spent as the vision of Mary came back to me, as she had begun that morning to tackle the daunting task of working her way back to some kind of normality again for the third time in 20 years.

But when I returned mid-afternoon, it seemed that the effort she had put into it all, no doubt for the benefit of all three of us, had proved too much for her, and she had wilted like some delicate, exotic plant put out into a biting wind.

By the next morning she seemed to have largely recovered again, and during the rest of that week showed further small but significant signs of improvement. She began to say a few more words, like "Hullo," and "All right" (the latter sometimes a somewhat grudging agreement to take some fluid after I had impressed on her the importance of doing so – she made it plain in her tone of voice what she thought of my persistence!).

On the Friday, a week after the stroke, I took her flowers purchased with money sent by her brother. A nurse was with us as I gave her the flowers and explained that they were from "Eric", and she immediately turned to the nurse and said very plainly, "My brother."

Unless one has experienced being cut off in this way from someone one is very close to, there is no knowing the music on the ear which two simple words like that can be.

In the meantime, my enthusiasm for keeping up Mary's fluid intake knew no bounds, and by the end of Saturday morning I had managed to get her to imbibe among other things a couple of fruit Yoghurts and a Gooseberry Fool (the latter one of her great favourites).

A major contingent from the family turned up at lunchtime, led by John and Roger, the idea being that subsequently we would all go out to lunch together whilst Mary was taking her rest.

It became a very belated lunch, for by the time we were ready to go, Mary seemed in great distress, and it was very difficult to leave her in such a state without knowing what was troubling her. Again, there is no describing the experience unless you have been there yourself; but in the end I had to leave her, still not knowing what was wrong.

When I returned later that afternoon she seemed quite alright again, and I was greeted by a wry smile from one of the nurses. She said, simply, "Try not to give your wife too many Gooseberry Fools in future!"

Despite my over-enthusiasm with the likes of Gooseberry Fool, Mary was reported as having had a very good sleep that night, and when I arrived after breakfast on Sunday morning she was absolutely wonderful. She was already up and dressed, and sitting in her chair, her face bright and smiling as I turned into the bay. There was, at once, a feeling of transformation in the air – as though something had 'clicked into place', so to say, and changed everything. She tried herself out on a whole lot of new words – not very successfully, but fresh effort and enthusiasm had seemingly sprung from nowhere. How well I remembered from 20 years before

> ... that little burble
> Interspersed
> With laughter –

> And what matter
> That meanings sometimes went astray
> In wordless chatter? –
> What matter?
> Oh! how we met!

It is possible that the improvement she showed that Sunday morning would in any event have proved a flash in the pan – that will never be known for certain – but ever since that day I have been tempted to think tragically otherwise.

It was the weekend, remember, when the ward had largely to run itself, with little or no high-level supervision or help, except in the case of an emergency. And there was a sense in which Mary's sudden and spectacular improvement was itself an emergency, as much in need of that high-level help and advice as any life-threatening one would have been.

The nurse in charge was the one with whom I had had the brush ten days earlier, concerning the dressing on Mary's ankle ulcer. She was her usual bustling self, still needing to prove something, still anxious to exercise as conspicuously as maybe the authority vested in her. The combination of such a trait with the circumstances obtaining in the ward at a weekend was potentially a dangerous one, and even now, as I write, over three years on, it is difficult to persuade myself that it did not at least hasten Mary's end. There was no question of negligence, just a surfeit of enthusiasm, combined with a monolithic attitude to the wielding of vested power and authority. And, to redress the balance still further, let it be said that this particular nurse was one of the very first to come and try to comfort me, just after Mary had died.

What happened then, that fateful Sunday morning, when I had found myself so unexpectedly on Cloud Nine?

The nurse's response to the sudden change in Mary was at once both dramatic and drastic. Until then, since the stroke, Mary had stayed quietly in the armchair by her bedside, out of sight and range of the hustle and bustle of the day-room, with all its comings and goings. But no sooner had the nurse recognised the quite spectacular improvement in Mary, than she immediately ordered her to be wheeled off to the day-room. She gave no reasons, but I would imagine that the decision was based on the belief that the response to any sign of progress should be to apply immediate pressure to produce still more. There seemed to be no recognition in such a philosophy of the need for, and the benefits of, consolidation. 'Press on regardless' was the order of the day, with no appreciation of the need to 'Hurry up slowly.'

Merely to spend the morning in the day-room, instead of by her bedside, might have made little or no difference to Mary, since I was to be with her, and we had our own ways of remaining fairly oblivious to our surroundings when we were together. It was what happened after that that did the damage, I believe.

Instead of being allowed to go back to her bedside again at lunchtime, and my being able to give her some of the little pots of 'slip-down-easy' food I had been feeding her with all week, it was insisted that Mary should sit up at table with all the others, and try to eat the ordinary food as best she could – 'cruel to be kind' is as good a gloss as can be put on it.

In the event, and after nearly an hour on the part of a nursing auxiliary spent trying to get even a few mouthfuls of food into Mary they gave up, and came and asked me (I had been waiting anxiously on the concourse) if I would try.

Poor Mary – she was utterly exhausted by the time I was called in to help, and I could get nowhere with her, though I tried for another half hour or so. Gone was the opportunity to feed her with anything at all for the time being – even one of those little egg custards – and I went to the nurse and said as much, at the same time reminding her that Mary rested on her bed for two hours in the afternoon, and thinking to myself as I did so of how much she would need that rest, in the circumstances. I said that I had to go and get a bite of lunch myself, and would be back again at teatime, after Mary's rest.

I was late getting back, for I had been late leaving. It didn't seem to me to matter much, as Mary would have been safely back on her bed, and resting for most of that time. Or so I thought.

But she was not on her bed when I got back, and not in her armchair either. I found her in a gaggle of armchairs in the day-room, engulfed in a crowd of other patients and their Sunday afternoon visitors, and in a virtually collapsed state. I asked the first nurse I could set eyes on whether Mary had had her rest. She looked blank, and said that she didn't know she had to have one. Apparently, after the exhausting time of the lunch-hour fiasco, Mary had spent the whole afternoon on her own amidst the hassle of the day-room, when she so desperately needed to be resting on her bed.

Following my intervention, they put her to bed there and then, in the early evening. But it was too late to prevent the day from being a catastrophe for her: simply because she had shown such singular improvement that morning, she had been kept up in the day-room for eight or nine hours, and expected to make a good showing at eating normal food again – yes, just like that. In such a situation there is no point in attempting to lay blame ("It is given only to God to know why anything happens"), and in the last analysis the nurse concerned was probably as much a victim of her own circumstances as Mary was of hers.

The remainder of that evening was spent with Mary, trying, on and off, to get a little nourishment into her, to take the place of what she had missed at lunchtime. In the end, she did have a little egg custard, and a little ice cream, and last thing I managed to get her to take a cup of Horlicks, but it amounted almost to force-feeding her. Part of the way through it, desperately anxious, I said, "You must drink this, it is so important." And at the very end of a disastrous day, which had begun with such promise, she gave me my reward – just four words, but spoken so plainly, "All right, I will."

I was not told what sort of night Mary had had after that terrible Sunday, but when I arrived after breakfast on the Monday morning the contrast with the previous morning was horrifying. Again the image of a wilting plant reared itself in my mind's eye, but added to it now was a strange air of preoccupation. As I sat chatting, trying to capture her interest, she was staring round the ward unhearing, looking first at this, then at that, sometimes as though she had never seen it before, and at other times, it seemed, with apprehension, as in a nightmare, almost as though she was expecting some strange and frightening apparition to appear. It was behaviour I had never seen before in her, and given my long conditioning regarding even the slightest change, I was puzzled and inexplicably perturbed by it.

In the middle of all this the consultant arrived, to begin his round of Mary's bay. My presence as the only visitor so early in the day would have made it difficult for him to ignore me, anyway, but the thought of what Mary had been like only twenty-four hours before, compared with her strange mood that morning, and the bad impression it might make on him, gave me the courage I needed, and goaded me into gate-crashing his ward round.

Far from brushing me off as a mere layman (as he might well have done), he took me very seriously indeed, and for a few minutes I might well have been one of his party, much to the discomfiture of the nurse responsible for the misadventures of the day before. There was no way in which I could avoid all reference to what had gone on, but I kept it in as general terms as possible, describing to him in some detail how magnificent Mary had been to begin with, and how the day's regimen had exhausted her, so that, among other things, she had been unable to take as much food or fluid as she had on the

Saturday. Mary had perked up with his arrival, and actually even smiled a little mischievously, like a naughty schoolgirl, as I told him of some of the difficulties I was having in getting her to take her food and drink.

He thanked me for what I was doing, asking me to "carry on with the good work", and winding up with the practical advice that whatever I gave her should be as cold as possible, ice-cold if possible, since that would stimulate the swallow reflex.

All this time the nurse in charge looked on, not a little out of countenance, even looking somewhat frustrated that her decisions of the day before should have been challenged, albeit obliquely, in this way.

Soon afterwards a young physiotherapist turned up, and did some passive physiotherapy with Mary, which only served to emphasise the terrible contrast with the first week, when Mary had walked on my arm down the concourse so that they could assess what, if anything, was wrong with her caliper. How quickly our attitudes are changed! Then, I was worried about Mary's walking, wondering what their assessment of it would be – but that Monday morning, as the physiotherapist strove to get even the simplest of responses from Mary's legs as she lay flopped on the bed, I would have settled for that walking so thankfully, the little hobble and all.

After the physiotherapist had gone Mary took a 5oz pot of yoghurt and 3fl oz of water in some sort of fashion; and later, at her lunchtime, a 6oz egg custard and a further 4oz of water. Optimistically, I duly made the corresponding entries on her fluid chart – "optimistically" because I was never quite sure how much of what I managed to put into her mouth actually trickled out of the side of it again and got absorbed in her bib. These entries on the chart were beginning to relate more to my own comfort and satisfaction than to hard reality.

This particular feeding session had been difficult for both of us, and at the end of it I said to Mary that I really had to go then to get a bite of lunch for myself, or I would probably, as I put it, "sink through the floor." And to my amazement, she gave me a real little giggle, by way of a reply. She was so game.

Whenever I left Mary's bed on the way out, I had to pass one of the men's bays, and I had become friendly with a young man whose late middle-aged father had been admitted for general nursing care following a fall downstairs. There didn't seem to have been any serious damage done, and certainly no broken bones. The two of them lived together, the father widowed, the son an only child, and he was desperately concerned about his father's fall. I remember succumbing to a tinge of envy the week before, as I compared his father's age with Mary's, and the relative lack of seriousness of his accident, compared with Mary's stroke. This had been followed by a strong sense of fellow feeling when he had told me one day that he was having great difficulty in getting his father to take his food. He was as worried about his father (unnecessarily I thought, at the time) as I was about Mary, and he began to spend as much time as I did at the hospital – which meant all his time, apart from his own meal times. The fellow feeling became mutual, and deepened steadily with the exchange of news about our respective patients whenever we met.

I asked him how his father was, and he told me that he had developed pneumonia. He was shattered, and I tried to comfort him, saying that his father was relatively young, and that modern antibiotics were so effective. He looked pathetically grateful for the encouragement, but turned away, and went back to his vigil.

Under stress, one's mind tends to be like a ship, with its watertight bulkheads which can be sealed off from one another, to prevent the contents of one compartment from invading another. Strokes were strokes, and pneumonia was pneumonia, and at least Mary hadn't got an acute illness like that to cope with – or so I thought, that Monday lunchtime.

The afternoon and evening were much the same as the morning had been. There was that same strange and peculiar air of preoccupation about Mary, as she sat in the armchair by her bed, gazing round at the other occupants of the bay, and at the comings and goings of the ward staff. It was almost as though she had just arrived and was trying to make out what it was all about: I had the greatest of difficulty in getting her to pay any attention at all to the perpetual problems of food and fluid intake.

I always went back last thing in the evening, around 9 o'clock or so, when the final round with the drugs trolley was under way, and patients were being tucked up for the night. I needed to see Mary settled, and, if possible, to know that she had gone to sleep, before I left the hospital. That was the only way I could settle down for the night myself, once I was home again.

But Mary was restless, and rather than continue to be a possible distraction at her bedside, I went and sat on the concourse, within sight of her, so that I would be able to tell when she had finally gone off to sleep.

It got to half past ten, and the nurses came to me then, saying that Mary would be in good hands, and virtually ordering me to go, pointing out that I myself badly needed rest.

I went, reluctantly, and with heavy heart, feeling that there was something about the day, and Mary's strange behaviour, that I hadn't understood.

And if I had had any thought that a night's sleep was going to change things for Mary, I was to be gravely disappointed in the morning. When I went as usual after breakfast, it was to find her still in bed, and obviously very under the weather now. For most of the day she lay, propped up by her pillows, only occasionally opening her eyes, even whilst I was trying to feed her. A doctor who came to look at her briefly told me that the "pots of this and that" didn't matter now, but that the fluid was important, and during the rest of that day I managed to give her around 400ml of water, and most of two ice creams. But when I left in the early evening, after ward supper-time, it was with the growing realisation that quite apart from the aftermath of the stroke, Mary was becoming ill in quite another way.

I had my evening meal with Roger and Wendy, and shared my fears with them. I was beginning to feel that I couldn't trust my own impressions any longer, and said as much, and Roger offered to go back with me then at 9 o'clock, for my final visit of the day, so that there would be the benefit of a second opinion.

It was dusk when we arrived, and the main ward lights were already dimmed for the night as we approached Mary's bay. There were no nurses about: they were down the far end of the ward, busy with the drugs trolley.

It was yet another of those moments of sheer horror, the sound and the sight of it fixed for ever on memory's ear as well as mind's eye. Long before we reached Mary's bed we could hear the awful sound of her breathing. Afterwards, we came to know that so characteristic was this sound, and so specific its diagnostic significance, that it had been given a name of its own, based on the names of two early nineteenth century physicians, who had observed and documented it. I was blissfully ignorant of both the name and its significance, as I tore along the concourse to seek out the drugs trolley, and its attendant nurses.

One of them, looking suddenly very serious, came back with me at once. She stopped for just a moment by Mary's bedside, just long enough to say, "That is Cheyne-Stokes breathing," adding immediately, "I must get a doctor." Contrary to my ill-founded belief of only the day before – that it was something she wouldn't have to cope with – Mary, in fact, had pneumonia.

Again a flood of questions. How long had she been like that? What difference had that made? – and how much longer might it have been before her condition was discovered, had Roger and I not gone back for my usual bedtime visit? Half an hour? An hour? What effect might that have had?

And the events of those last three days, apparently disparate and unrelated, began to fall into place, like the parts of a jigsaw that, seemingly having borne no relationship to one another, are suddenly seen to be the component parts of a coherent picture: Sunday, when the ill-considered over-enthusiasm of a nurse led to the virtual exhaustion of Mary by the end of the day; Monday, and the sudden withdrawal of Mary's energies and her relative inability to cope with her surroundings any longer; and Tuesday, the onset of rampant pneumonia.

Chapter Eighteen

The doctor they found that Tuesday night was a young woman, who, with her limited amount of training and experience, did her best to cope with the situation in which she found herself – that of dealing with me at that time of night, as well as with Mary.

She took me on one side, and said baldly, bleakly, "Your wife may well not survive the night."

The conditioning of 20 years rose to the surface then, and I found myself declaring for the second time in those 20 years, and with the same vehemence that I had used in 1978, "*My wife is a survivor.*"

Together we had won so many battles, major and minor ones alike, that I had come dangerously near to believing that Mary would always survive whatever life flung at her.

Despite this, as Roger and I watched over her in the small hours of that night, I found myself briefly contemplating the ultimate – of Mary *not* surviving, and the repercussions of that for myself. There had been those who, immediately on hearing that Mary had had yet another stroke, had (in effect) whispered, "You must let her go now. She has had enough, and so have have you, too. It is time."

I had understood what was being said, and that nothing but kindness had motivated it, but I well remember responding to one such firmly expressed opinion with the equally firm statement that I was "incapable of looking in two directions at once": I knew that it would be impossible to do all that was within my power to fulfil Mary's cheery parting remark to our homely help, "See you again soon," and at the same time to be deliberately planning for a new life without her. Nevertheless, the seed thought had been sown, and, for a few moments, in the weariness of the night watches, it came back to haunt and (must I say it in the good, old-fashioned way?) to tempt me with the thought that perhaps, after all, Mary herself (if she could have done) would have said that she had had enough. For a brief instant the prospect of us both being freed from the bondage of her handicaps held me, but a mere moment later, and it came to me that, given only one wish for the rest of my life, it would most certainly have been for Mary to get well enough to be able to enjoy her life again, and for me to be able to look after her once more.

Thus did that night's vigil serve its unanticipated purpose – that of clarifying just where I stood with Mary, and that, in turn, produced a great peace of mind for me during what did, in fact, turn out to be the last days of her life.

They had given Mary an injection of antibiotic, and put her on a drip; and within a very few hours we were able to observe her breathing becoming normal again. By the morning I felt my faith in Mary completely vindicated: for she had survived.

We left before breakfast, and I managed two hours sleep before going back again. Mary was up but not dressed, in her armchair by her bed, wearing that strange, 'preoccupied' look again, as though she no longer quite belonged to her surroundings. Whatever state of mind it was, it seemed to apply to everything, including my attempts to feed her, and to get fluid into her. She seemed to be barely able to attend to anything. From time to time, though, there were bouts of frustration or anger (it was impossible to tell which), fuelling the sense of a brewing crisis, despite the fact that she had survived the night. The inability to discern what was troubling her and thus to be able to do something about it was an agony in itself, which grew to fill the whole morning.

She wouldn't (or couldn't?) open her mouth even once to take any food, and there I had to leave it, at 1.30, when they came to put her back to bed. Home then, perhaps to rest a bit myself, before going back mid-afternoon.

Nothing had changed. Mary was fretful and frustrated from time to time, though she did manage to sleep a little, in between. I was desperate to get at least some fluid into her, and teaspoonful by teaspoonful, I did manage to spoon in about 120ml or so. But she didn't really swallow it. It just 'gurgled' down; and how much of it left again by the other side of her mouth was impossible to tell. The entry of 120ml on her fluid chart was so much wishing thinking, and for my own comfort, rather than as any statement of fact.

The food trolley came round, and, as other patients, able freely to express their choice in words, were being served up with hearty suppers, I fell victim for a few moments to a combination of simple envy and resentment. I imagined what it would be like to able to accept a whole plateful of food like that for Mary, and to feed it to her, as we chatted of this and that. Throughout her illnesses, I would from time to time fall for such fantasies, only to have to recognise them for what they were, and to come back with a jolt to the harsh realities again.

Recollecting, then, the advice of the consultant about ice-cold food, and with a strange feeling that the food trolley was of another world, to which Mary and I no longer belonged, I went up to it and asked the nurse if I could have an ice cream for Mary, almost as though it was some special concession. But it was of no use – she took little or nothing of it, and I had to leave again, taking comfort from the fact that she had maintained a reasonably normal breathing pattern all day, but all too aware that there was something which was troubling her, the nature of which I had failed completely to understand. It was my turn, then, to be overwhelmed by frustration.

When I got back to the ward again at 9 o'clock, for my bedtime visit, it was to find them changing Mary's catheter, which at some time during the day had apparently become blocked. One didn't need to look any further for the cause of poor Mary's discomfort, and one was faced with yet another example of the consequences of under-staffing. The devotion of the nurses was total, but each of them could be in one place only at a time, had only one pair of eyes with which to discern a need, and only one pair of hands with which to meet it.

Mary's breathing, though a little 'bubbly and squeaky' and a trifle fast, was still quite regular, and during that last visit for the day we had really good and meaningful eye contacts again, which were a great comfort. I felt that she had come back again, after the Monday and the Tuesday, when, it seemed, she had been so preoccupied with a far land.

And that Wednesday night, July 6th, I slept in my own bed again, with a somewhat easier mind.

The recollection of the next seven days is incomplete, and blurred – probably because they were all much the same as each other, and unmarked by any further great crisis. Mary was on a continuous drip, so that for the time being there wasn't the problem of fluid intake to worry about, although, increasingly, the nursing staff were exercised to find fresh sites for the drip: Mary's arms were becoming peppered with the appearance of small bruises which each new site produced. With the aid of the little pots of egg custard and the like, I continued to try to stimulate her swallow reflex, and to get some ordinary nourishment into her, but a new and almost uncanny quality began to envelop my visits to the ward. It was to do with time, as though time was slowing up for us, as though we were in a sort of backwater all to ourselves, whilst the rest of the world went by, in its own time flux, unchanged.

One morning during that period, I arrived after breakfast to find Mary propped up in bed and looking as radiant as an angel. Indeed, I remember using some such words to describe to our GP how she was that morning. All the stress lines had left her features, and she looked suddenly thirty years younger. Strangely, it seemed, he did not appear to share my enthusiasm. I did not ask him why, and I have never followed up the matter since, but I realise now that to his medical mind it was not a good sign at all. Such is the bliss that ignorance so often brings.

In the event, it all appeared to be a mere lull, which presaged yet another storm. Mary's breathing began to get very difficult again, though there was never a return to the awfulness of the Cheyne-Stokes pattern. Once again I was taken into the doctor's room, off the ward, and told, not simply that Mary might not survive the night, but that she almost certainly would not do so.

By now my belief in her immortality was almost total, and I protested even more vehemently than I had done the week before that she was a survivor, and that I believed she would once again survive. The doctor, another woman, but a more senior one this time – probably a registrar – looked at me kindly, but her disagreement was all too evident in her features.

Once again Roger and I stayed through the night with Mary, and once again she was with us still, in the morning. The doctor came early on, and with a frankly baffled look, she said, quite simply, "You were right, weren't you?"

The pneumonia, though, was taking its toll of Mary's strength. She lay for long periods with her eyes shut, and there was little I could do except to keep vigil over her.

Indeed, there seemed to be less and less that anyone could do for her. Not only that, but as I look back on that time I realise now, in fact, that those in overall charge of her were already beginning to shed some of the burden of treatment, on her behalf. For my part I could not (or would not?) recognise the significance of some of the things that were said, and done, at the time.

For example, there was a ward round that day, and I took the opportunity to express my concern over the fact that, owing to the very great difficulty in getting her to take her pills, Mary was falling behind with her routine drugs. I was merely told that her blood pressure was not untowardly high, and so, not to bother her with the pills. I distinctly remember feeling that here, at least, was something to be grateful for – that for the time being, at any rate, she was able to do without those 'sixteen-inch gun' drugs she had been taking for so long.

For some reason, too, they took her off her drip, only restoring it, I am tempted to think now, to placate the untoward anxiety which I began to show about it. Increasingly, a feeling of extemporisation crept into their treatment of Mary, decisions looking more and more ad hoc, and made from hour to hour, often with the appearance of quite arbitrary changes of direction. It was as though the overall battle strategy had been abandoned, and decisions relating to Mary were being taken by the field commanders.

We struggled through in this way to Saturday, July 16th, which I have good reason to remember as the day of the Hospital Fete.

I suppose that in my heart of hearts I was aware that things were getting more and more difficult, not only for Mary herself, but also for those responsible for her nursing care. Perhaps, too, the combination of these two things was making me paranoic on Mary's behalf. Subconsciously, I was refusing to recognise that the lack, now, of any hustle and bustle round Mary's bed meant simply that there was little left that they could do for her, apart from easing any pain or discomfort; and I was beginning to transmute my fears for Mary into a mute accusation of neglect by the hospital staff – a classic psychological side-step, if ever there were one.

And what better event to feed such a misapprehension than a Hospital Fete? I had arrived back after lunch, and the fete was already in full swing on the sports field below Mary's window. The contrast between what was going on outside the window, and what was going on inside, as I desperately tried, teaspoonful by teaspoonful, to get Mary to take some water, could hardly have been more dramatic.

But the issue was finally pointed (so it seemed, at the time) when I went to enter the amount on Mary's fluid chart. It wasn't there. I marched up to the desk and asked for it, assuming that it had been removed temporarily for entering the record in Mary's notes. The nurse didn't have it, either. Where was it?, I asked. She didn't know, and whoever it was who was responsible for making out another one was at the fete, she said, but she promised me she would get a new one made out, directly they were back.

I am sure now, as I think about it again, that deep down I knew that we were playing a game of charades – going through the motions on my behalf – and that really the time and the need for records of fluid intake were past, for Mary. But I was still not able to admit any such thing to myself, and grudgingly, and somewhat ungraciously, I accepted the promise of a new chart, as soon as it could be arranged.

It duly appeared at the foot of Mary's bed in the early evening, and I, in my turn, went through the motions of entering the minuscule amount of water which I had been able to get Mary to take.

This episode of the fluid intake chart may well have set the stage for the next, and fateful day of Sunday, July 17th, exactly one month after Mary had been admitted to hospital.

I had not long arrived in the ward when I was approached by a staff nurse whom I had never seen before. I was immediately struck by the fact that her appearance was belied by her manner. She was probably in her middle 30s, a tall and very well-built woman – taller than me, and certainly weighing a lot more – but she could not have been kinder or gentler in her manner, and in the way she treated me. I sensed at once that the kindness and the gentleness were born of a very great deal of understanding of where I stood that morning, and of the dire need to fulfil the task which she had been given – nothing less than convincing me that Mary was dying, indeed, that she would die within the next 24 hours.

Why was it that I didn't protest any longer that Mary was a survivor? It wasn't, I am quite sure, simply because the nurse had convinced me, out of her expertise, and with the weight of her experience, that there was no gainsaying the matter this time. No, it wasn't that. In fact, and on the contrary, it was because she hadn't spoken merely in such terms that I was able to take from her what I had been unable to accept from the two doctors, earlier. Although she spoke unemotionally, and, to a casual observer, even in a very matter-of-fact manner, I knew that in her spirit she had joined me, where I was, so that, in that moment of truth, I was not alone. It was not 'all in a day's work for her': for those few minutes she was with me, in my agony.

Thus it was that she enabled me to find myself again, and to be able to pick up the phone, and in a straightforward way to appraise our family and a handful of close friends of the situation.

All the family in turn came to the hospital that afternoon, and Roger brought a little bag of sandwiches for us both, so that we could stay on through the night, without having to seek out food for ourselves.

I had been told by the nurse that Mary would not be in any appreciable pain, and though I asked no questions, I presumed that that meant a modicum of morphine, to ease her into that milieu of the spirit where she would be free at last of the burden of all her disabilities.

The nurses had settled Mary down for the night, and she was as comfortable as they could make her. Her breathing was regular, but rapid, and terribly fluid-laden. They would come during the night to relieve that, with a sort of aspirator, wheeled in on a trolley – a contraption which in that situation seemed little short of fiendish. It seemed so clumsy and so crude, to have Mary subjected to its attentions in the small hours when, in another order, and some other dispensation, she could have been tucked up in her own bed at home, and sound asleep. It all began to take on the quality of nightmare.

Her eyes were closed, either in light and restless sleep, or a semi-conscious condition – it was impossible to tell which – and we settled down as best we could for the long vigil. There was no question of sleep, except for the brief snatches to which tired bodies and exhausted spirits would inevitably succumb for a few minutes, from time to time. One woke from these with a sense of disbelief; and as the reality was borne in upon one anew, it brought with it the awful feeling of having abandoned Mary to her fate, albeit so briefly, and out of sheer frailty of mind and body ("Could you not watch with me one hour?").

There was no way of knowing whether Mary was conscious of our physical presence in those last hours of her life, but I believe that even if she was unaware of us through the agency of her five senses, her spirit, for sure, would have known that there were those who loved and cherished her, who were keeping vigil with her.

She managed to soldier on into the dawn, and there followed an uneasy and restless two or three hours before the nurses suddenly appeared in strength round her bed, soon after 7am, ostensibly to wash and tidy her, and sort out the bed. They shooed us off to the day room whilst this was going on, but we had been there hardly a moment when one of them came hurrying back to us.

"Come quickly!" was all she said.

We ran along the concourse to the bay where Mary was, and arrived at her bedside just seconds before she died. I cannot use the usual cliché and say that she died totally peacefully, for it seemed to me that right until her very last breath she struggled for the oxygen which would keep her alive, and amongst us still.

As that last breath left her body, I gently closed her unseeing eyes, and left her bedside immediately.

I had seen many dead people in my life, but it so happened that never before had I seen anyone actually die. Why did Mary have to be the very first? – Mary, the one with whom my whole life had become so inextricably involved, through daily and hourly attendance upon her.

That last gasp of hers might very well have been seen to be my last gasp, too. For I also had to die to the old life, the life in which my very identity had become so largely vested in Mary's care. But it was to prove a lingering and very painful death, and one which, over three years on, is still in process.

Epilogue

Chapter Nineteen

Let me
At least take comfort
From my tears –
That there is yet left
Enough of me
To weep,
Not simply, now, for loss of you,
But for a myriad
Unacknowledged pains
Deep buried
By the wayside
Of our journey
Through those stricken years.

"I weep,
Therefore I am" –
Thus do I reassure myself
That desolation
Has not laid final waste
To me;
Yet
On that journey
Did I, like those
In heat of battle smitten,
Soldier on,
Unaware
That when the strife was at an end
I would have mortal wounds
To tend.

Weep then,
Scan the bleak landscape
Of those fraught, fateful years,
Drink the full draught
Of unassimilated pain,
And the then unshed,
Countless tears.

I had joined the U3A – "The University of the Third Age", a rapidly growing organization for the over-50s, providing study and discussion groups on all sorts of topics, ranging from modern languages to photography, art to opera, and history to current affairs. I had already joined a painting class run by a private art school, but my family thought that a few more regular activities would provide a framework round which I could begin to build a new life. I joined the Current Affairs Group, which met in a room let to the organization by a small convent. It was my very first attendance.

The room was modern, and pleasantly furnished, and all round it were large wall posters, excellent reproductions of colour photographs, each of which had been given an appropriate caption. I was almost the first to arrive, and spent the time going round the room, studying the posters. As George Fox would have said, they very much "spoke to my condition". One was particularly memorable. It was a photograph taken from inside a sea cavern, looking out onto a sunlit sea. The blackness of the cave walls served only to enhance the brilliance of the sunlit scene beyond. The caption ran something like, "Beyond the darkness, the light".

At that moment those words struck a deep chord in me, as did the words on a number of the other posters. I heard little of the discussion that morning, far too busy with my own current affairs.

We had been served with coffee and biscuits by the nuns, and on the way out at the end of the morning, I passed the open kitchen door, and could see one of them washing up. She happened to look my way, and acting on an impulse I began, falteringly, and near to tears, to say how much I had appreciated the posters. She asked me then, quite simply, what was troubling me, and I told her in a sentence or two of Mary, and of her death eight months before, and found myself saying what I had said so many times during that period – that I had not only lost Mary, but my whole role in life as well.

And what did she do? Quote me a text? (you know – "Blessed are they that mourn", and so on). Preach me a neat little homily? No – not at all! She flung her arms round me, gave me a whacking kiss on the lips, and said, simply, "What you need is a little love." The dammed-up tears, which "a little love" had released in me, began to flow then, and as I tried to hide them she said, "Jesus wept – please don't be afraid or ashamed to cry."

She had just time to ask me my name, and to say that she would remember me in her prayers, before I turned and fled. I needed to get home as quickly as possible, and drove straight off, despite the tears: they lasted the two or three-mile journey home, and for a full hour after it. It was during that time that "Let me at least take comfort..." was written.

Thus began a process of catharsis – of drinking "the full draught of unassimilated pain" – which has continued ever since, in a variety of forms – the latest of which is, indeed, this piece of writing.

Looking back, I realise now that the process had actually begun within days of Mary's dying, though many things, sad to say, had conspired to interrupt it. And it had started at the right place: at the very beginning of it all, with the pain – unassimilated even after twenty years – of finding Mary unconscious, in a coma, as I clutched the poem which was my vision of the future for us, but which was never to be realised – not in this life, anyway.

It had been a devastating moment, spiritually as well as emotionally, but as I read the poem over and over again in the immediate aftermath of Mary's death, I began to see in it an entirely new aspect and relevance.

> What does it matter,
> But that I meet thee now?
> My being with yours,
> Finding each other,
> And ourselves,
> Anew,
> After the long day's heat....

It came to me then that "the long day's heat" was no longer the arduous time we had spent bringing up a family, but was to be seen as those twenty years in which we both of us had been in bondage to Mary's disabilities. Released from that bondage at the moment of Mary's death, our two spirits were no longer inextricably tied in with each other: could not we, once more two separate beings, find each other, and ourselves, anew, in that separateness?

There was fresh hope in such a thought, and it quickly became linked with another insight I had had.

I had begun to suffer feelings of panic from time to time – feelings that the situation was intolerable, that Mary's death was something beyond my capacity to bear. These feelings mostly arose soon after putting out the light at night, or in the small hours, if I should happen to wake then. Well do I remember the prayer that I would use at such a moment, so near was it to the limit of what I could stand: "Lord help me to be just able to bear this unbearable thing, just able to tolerate this intolerable thing, just able to suffer this insufferable thing." To be just able to cope would be miracle enough, and there seemed to be no point in praying for more.

There was a night when, only half awake, I thought for a moment that I could hear Mary breathing beside me. I woke myself right up then, and in the panic that followed I started in my usual fashion to walk through the house from room to room, in a state of utmost agitation. Suddenly, I remembered that on that particular night, before going to bed, I had loaded both the washing machine and the dishwasher, and set them going; and by the time the panic was upon me, they had done their work for the night. I made a profound discovery then – which was simply to divert the otherwise uncontrollable, volcanic energy of the panic into a practical activity. I emptied the dishwasher, deliberately taking my time over it, putting each separate piece away carefully, where it belonged. Then I did the same thing with the washing, slowly folding each article, making neat piles, and finally stowing them away in the airing cupboard. All this took quite a long time, and I followed it by stripping my bed completely, and remaking it with fresh linen: I was no stranger to changing beds in the small hours. And at the end of all this the panic had subsided. Moreover, as a bonus, I had a nice, freshly-made bed to climb back into, when I was ready.

Another thing I was prompted to do that night before finally going back to bed, was to put the front door lock on the latch, so that anyone could let themselves in, if need be. This also had a calming effect: I felt less trapped inside the house, and thus less trapped inside myself.

Somehow or other, I had used the panic to do a number of jobs which, if I had got up at the normal time and tackled them, would have seemed really irksome. Their very irksomeness had completely vanished in the process – surely, good out of evil.

As, at long last, I made to get into bed again, I became aware of how thin the ice had been that I had skated on that night.

In fact, in quieter moments, I began to see the panics as nothing less than a crisis of identity. For years my life had been totally taken up with caring for Mary in her state of disability, and all that stemmed from it. But now the disabilities were no more, and the life which I had built round them had no reality any longer, either. Yet, I was still trying to hang on to that identity, mourning its very loss, even though Mary's life, and her disabilities with it, was at an end.

As this new-found separateness was borne in upon me, I began to realise that Mary certainly would not want me to go on clinging to that old life, or the identity associated with it; less still, to mourn its passing.

I had to start again, becoming nothing less than an entirely 'new man'; but I was to discover that that was to be no easy matter. Many times there were tantalising glimpses of what it would be like when I had achieved it, but, in Harry Williams' words again, "It hurts when the manacles which chain us to the past are broken" – I had to suffer the pain of dying to the old self, and then of being born into that new self which was waiting. I believe now that those "tantalising glimpses" were gifts of grace, when, for a moment, a minute or two, an hour, or blessedly but rarely for most of a day it was given to me to know, with Julian of Norwich, that "all shall be well, and all manner of thing shall be well".

In the meantime, wandering as in a maze through the wilderness of emotions that we call bereavement, I knew for the first time the depths plumbed by the experience. Never again could I watch, detached, as a reporter on the 'box', concerned only with the 'news-worthiness' of a story, blandly asked someone what it felt like to have just lost a spouse or a child in some tragedy or other, from a rare illness to a motorway pile-up, or a terrorist bomb. News-gathering can be almost as cruel as the event itself, and perhaps at its most cruel in its dealings with those just bereaved. I used to wonder what I would have answered when asked 'what it felt like'. Whatever the answer might have been, I hope that it would have created an awareness that reporters pushed their way into places where angels fear to tread, and would have made the offender think more than twice in the future, before posing such a question again.

As I look back, with insight born of hindsight, I realise that there were key moments, and key experiences, some of them very early on indeed, which, if I had properly grasped their significance at the time, would have greatly shortened the length of my journey through that wilderness. There was, for instance, Neville Ward's book, *Friday Afternoon*, to which I was introduced within weeks of Mary's death. The book is a series of meditations on Christ's last words from the cross, and deals in great depth and with great sensitivity with the experience of failure, and loss, and in particular, bereavement. I remember reading the book almost at a single sitting; and well on into it, inconspicuously embedded in the text, there was a brief paragraph which spoke volumes to me, rang all sorts of bells with me, but I seemed powerless at the time to take it to heart, and to act upon it: only now, over three years on, am I beginning to be able to do so. Says Neville Ward:

> There is a better and a worse way of dealing with disaster. However great the good of which life has been robbed by it, *new good* [italics mine] begins to be made if we choose the better way. There are powerful kinds of good that can come into life only where something has gone terribly wrong; it just happens to be one aspect of the composition of things. There is an Old Testament prayer, 'It is good for me that I have been in trouble, that I may learn thy law'.

> Neville Ward comments,

> There is more in it than that our mistakes at any rate serve to point out and underline the right way. The writer may have discovered this subtle principle of man's emotional and spiritual life – *the curious bonus attached to good that is erected forthwith on the actual site of failure and loss.* [Italics again mine.] (p.97)

> There were many other passages which, again with George Fox, I knew 'spoke to my condition', but which I seemed powerless to act

upon at the time. There was a quotation from Gabriel Marcel's book, *Homo Victor*: "it is never a simple return to the status quo, a simple return to our being, it is that and much more, and even the contrary of that: an undreamed-of promotion, a transfiguration." Neville Ward goes on later to comment, "Another word for this is 'resurrection'."

And there was that other wonderful thought, "Bereavement is loving in a new key." But I just couldn't cope with that either, at the time.

However, there was an experience, a crucial one, to which I was able to respond, and which has meant so much to me, ever since.

Five days after Mary's funeral, and with a thunderstorm threatening, I threw my painting gear into the car, and drove off into the country. I had no idea whether I would ever want to paint again, or, for that matter, whether I would still be able to; and, symbolically enough, I had no idea where I was going, either.

The pending storm added its own urgency – I had to be quick in my choice of subject, if there was to be any time at all to paint. My unconscious was in the driving seat, and I had gone barely two miles along a favourite lane, hardly wide enough for two cars, before coming to a natural lay-by at the entrance to a field. I pulled in, and switched the engine off, and sat, immobile and irresolute, watching the gathering storm, and beginning to feel that it had been a mistake even to contemplate putting the matter to the test so soon after Mary's death. It was precisely the kind of mood in which, in the tradition of the countryside, one felt the simple need of a five-barred gate to lean upon – and I climbed out of the car and did just that.

From the distance came the lazy sound of a tractor trundling back and forth, lulling me into the state where the mind is quiescent, and the imagination alert. In the foreground was the golden ochre of a newly-harvested field, and beyond that the burnt sienna of an older stubble, beyond that again field upon field vanishing into the storm haze. And over it all was the lowering sky, its threat alleviated by a single, small patch of blue.

It was that patch of blue, more than anything else, which sent me scurrying back to the car for my painting gear. For me, at that moment, it spelled the promise at the heart of the storm, and before the storm burst, soft pastels had captured the sky and that patch of blue, together with the far and middle distance. There, there was a line of dense woodland, 'blacker than black' and impenetrable under its branches; but immediately below it, almost lurid in the storm light, was the brilliant yellow ochre of a ripe and as yet unmowed cornfield.

The storm was short and sharp, and the painting was finished within a couple of hours of first taking up position at the five-barred gate.

Despite the initial and grave misgivings, it had, in the event, been painted with a sense of utmost urgency; and though there would be no Mary to whom I could take it home, as I had done all my other paintings, there was a distinct feeling that unlike all the others, she had actually participated in this one.

The painting spoke of the richness of the harvest, even under the threat of storm, and as it came into being on the painting board, it spoke to me, above all else, of the richness of the harvest of love in Mary's life, the sense of which no storm could take away, even the storm of bereavement. And all who have shared this painting with me, including many who knew nothing of the circumstances in which it was painted, have said that there was something special about it. I believe that that was because Mary had actually taken part in it.

There were other occasions when Mary seems to have intervened. I am not speaking of visions or voices outside myself, but of mental images, and thoughts, and dreams, which were of such a nature, and so utterly contrary to my prevailing mood, that it would be quite impossible to attribute them to any kind of wish fulfilment.

There was the time when I had been visiting Mary's grave, some months after she had died. It was a dreadful, late afternoon in November, murky and misty, as I turned away from the grave, distraught, tears welling. Suddenly, into my mind, and without anything at all to prompt them, came the words, "Come Lloyd! Come Lloyd! It's not that bad!"

Had there been anyone with me, who knew me at all well, they would have deemed my mood just then as inconsolable, and would certainly not have had the courage to address me in any such words. In any case, once the words had injected themselves into my mind I associated them immediately, and unquestioningly, with Mary.

Again, one day, as I was arranging flowers on Mary's grave, I was thinking of how, through the agency of my own two hands, two feet, eyes, ears and speech, Mary could continue to 'dwell among us', and in the very thought itself I felt I was making the offering of my being to Mary's. Suddenly then, in my inner eye, I saw her so plainly – no vision this, just a mental image. She was sitting so quietly, deeply pensive, as though pondering the significance of the thought I had shared with her. She seemed to me like a child wanting to say 'Thank you' for a special present, but unable to find the words. Then, immediately afterwards, I was possessed of another thought – that in that moment there had been a giving of each to the other, anew. But even this second thought was overtaken, as, in my mind's eye, I contemplated the serenity of Mary's appearance, and it came to me that, above all else, *it had been a vision of the life of pure spirit.*

There was a similar moment, too, soon after I had started writing this book, and yet again it followed a visit to Mary's grave. Indeed, my mind was still juggling with a welter of words as I went and sat on a seat that looked past the grave to the beautiful countryside beyond; and suddenly, into the middle of my words came others, from elsewhere. Once more, they were foreign to my flow of thought, and once more, without question, I associated them with Mary.

"There is so much to look forward to, Lloyd, and not back."

The words were so totally out of kelter with my own, and, indeed, seemingly critical of what I had set myself to do here, in this writing. They certainly unsettled me. I had to go on – I knew that; but I would take serious account thenceforward of what Mary had seemed to be saying to me – that it must be not merely to indulge myself, or to wallow in the past: it must be a clearing of the decks, in fact, for all that Mary was wanting me to look forward to. And I felt, in that moment, that she didn't mean just in this life.

The dangers involved in our dealings with the past are well described by Christopher Bryant in *Jung and the Christian Way*, when he speaks of "a tendency to get bogged down in the past, to cling to it for dear life and so to be hindered from grasping the opportunities and embracing the tasks of the present. We cling in nostalgia to a happiness or security we once enjoyed and long for its recovery."

This, one might feel, is obvious enough, but with subtle insight he adds, "Paradoxically we cling not only to good and happy memories but to painful and humiliating ones ... experiences of inconsolable grief, experiences so full of anguish as to be repressed and forgotten, live on in the unconscious like an invisible cancer, consuming psychic energy and sapping the individual's ability to face the present and the future." Bryant goes on, "The practice of thanksgiving" (which he has defined earlier as "the acknowledgement of God in the awareness of the good and helpful factors in life") "fosters a healthy detachment from, a letting go of the past, for it links past experience with the present reality of God.... Where the individual has a genuine faith the painful wounds of the past *once recalled* [italics mine] can be healed by thanksgiving. For thanksgiving declares the believer's faith in God's infinitely resourceful presence even within evil, mitigating its effects and bringing good out of it." "Indeed," adds Bryant, "the power of God to redeem and draw good out of evil is at the very heart of the gospel.... Thanksgiving cannot of course change the past, but it can change its effects, *through faith and memory working together,* [italics again mine] by bringing the past into the present of God, where old wounds can be healed and life imprisoned can be set free."

That, indeed, was the task to which I had set my hand.

There were dreams too, some disturbing, some comforting; and perhaps the most comforting of all was the one I had recently, very close to the third anniversary of Mary's death.

The beginning of it found me with Mary, quietly happy and contented. But soon, I had to take her back to where she was living. It was late at night, and she had been busy (and so happy) in some kind of work in which she was involved. Her room needed attending to, and her bed wasn't properly made; and I said to her, so gently, "Shall I tidy your room, and make your bed for you, before I go?"

We were relating to each other so understandingly, acceptive of the fact that she was busy, and had to live there, whilst I was living somewhere else. We were so gentle towards each other in our acceptance of the situation, as we parted for the night. It was wonderful – Mary her old self, having none of her disabilities any longer, and full of a quiet energy and enthusiasm for what she was doing; and I, utterly content on her behalf, in spite of the fact that I had got to leave her again. We recognised that we each had things to do, which would keep us apart for the time being. There seems to have been a great symbolism in that – of the fact that Mary had died, and of our acceptance that for the time being we were living in two different orders and dispensations. As I contemplated the dream, I rejoiced that in it, despite our independent lives, we related to each other so maturely, and with such total accord.

Later that day on which I had woken from this dream it came back to me that before I had gone to bed the previous night my prayer had been that I might be given a new awareness of the presence of Mary's spirit with me.

Surely, the dream was the answer.

Chapter Twenty

Such occurrences, however, were, in truth, relatively isolated, with long barren stretches, and worse, in between. There was much inevitable self-scrutiny: if's and but's, and why's and wherefore's and if only's – the "Ash Wednesday" experience, as I came to think of it. I joined the sad company of those who, in TS Eliot's words, "walk in noise ... torn on the horn between season and season, time on time, between hour and hour, word and word, power and power", "wavering between the profit and the loss", until I longed to "forget these matters that with myself I too much discuss, too much explain"; longed to "care and not to care ... to sit still".

Of course there was some distortion of perspective in all this, and there were those among family and friends who did their best to straighten me out.

Our vicar, commenting on what he called "the remarkable fact of Mary's survival for 20 years", said that it probably had more than a little to do with the fact that she did feel so secure – and that was some comfort to me. And he added that perhaps she did have some inkling, too, of what her loss would mean to me, and that she soldiered on for as long as she did, in part, at any rate, to spare me that pain for as long as she could, even though it prolonged her suffering in this life. Certainly, that would have been very much within Mary's character to do just that.

And John, our older son, in the immediate agonising aftermath of Mary's death, pointed out that in whatever ways my care of her might have fallen short, what I had done for her had fulfilled my main hope – that she should never have to be institutionalised. I do realise that if that had had to be, it would have broken Mary's heart; and it would certainly have broken mine. As John pointed out so wisely, I had to accept the pain of bereavement as the price I would eventually have to pay, if Mary was to be spared that fate.

There was another, and more mystical comfort which I was given at that time.

Immediately after Mary's death, I turned to Harry Williams yet again, and re-read his little book, *Becoming What I Am*. It was at the time of the worst of my self-doubtings, and just as I was becoming aware that I had an identity crisis on my hands. Harry Williams is so good at advocating approaching God *just as you are* – no airs or graces, no pretensions. "... wherever I am, or whatever I am doing, whether I feel tired or excited, angry or amused, a bundle of nerves or calm and quiet, miserable or happy, optimistic or in despair, let me see," he says, "that all I have to do is to turn simply to God and say 'Hello, it is me.' And when you can do simply that," Harry Williams says so characteristically, "there is joy in heaven among the angels of God."

But, crucially, and indeed cryptically, he goes on to say that "Hello, it is me" "is an answer to a prayer as well as a prayer itself."

Now, there came one of those distraught days, when whatever I had done for Mary seemed to me to have dwindled into near-insignificance compared with what I might have done; and, close to despair, I took Harry Williams' advice, and simply said, "Hello God, this is me."

What happened then was a startling confirmation that "Hello, it is me" was a prayer capable of providing its own answer. For I had hardly uttered it when I had a seemingly totally incongruous mental vision of Mary and me on holiday in Abergavenny in 1986, the last proper holiday we had.

For the first time, in a flash of awareness, I saw the risks involved (albeit unwittingly) in such an undertaking. Quite apart from managing the ordinary mechanics of living, in a hotel, and away from our home base, I saw plainly for the first time the hazards of being out and about with someone as vulnerable as Mary was, perhaps on a lonely mountain road, or a mile or two into a dense woodland, on a single-width cart track miles from anywhere. Foolhardy? I don't know. What I do know, is that in that moment after I had said, in all the wretchedness of self-doubt, "Hello, God, it is me," it was as though, in that vision, God was saying to me, "Yes, this is you, but that was you, too."

Come to think of it, the test of any deep relationship should be the possibility of being able to say "Hello, this is me," – warts and all, no pretences, airs or graces – and to find oneself accepted.

But I was not without my 'comforters' of the ilk that offered Job the benefit of their wisdom – all good-intentioned, but unaware of the wilderness I still inhabited, most of the time.

Many said
That it was over now;
Others, that I should be thankful;
A few (I fear) that it was simply
God's will that had been done,
(Like the hurricane last year) –
But I knew the life, which,
In my heart,
Had only just begun.

Death gave it birth: your passing
The cosmic contraction
That propelled me
On the headfirst journey
Through the tortuous tunnel
Of fierce disbelief –
With pain beyond thought –
Into a future
Furnished
With an empty chair,
An empty bed,
Coats still hanging, ready,
In the hall;
Your place at table vacant,
Meal on meal.

Morning upon morning,
Listless and leaden-eyed
I lie,
Hoping the world
Will pass me by.
What chance of that? –
The harsh light of reality
Leaves no margin
For the re-interpretation
Of events;
Better to weep my way
Into the crevices
Of yet another day –
Others, perchance,
Will neither find
Nor even seek me
There.

But –
Tread warily;
At every twist and turn
Of time
And space
There lies in wait
Some devastating evocation
Of the past –
Beyond tears:
From a paper scrap,

With frail words
Traced by that rebellious hand,
To your first caliper, lurking
In the dark depths
Of a wardrobe
Where I sought
A long-lost pair of shoes.
(God alone knows
The volumes spoken
By a piece of bent iron
Fitted with a leather thong
And metal peg –
The vision, too,
That it evoked
Of you,
With your strapped leg
And walking frame,
And those first faltering steps -
God, indeed, alone knows
The courage that you showed.)

Beyond tears, yes,
But weep noneless;
Grief's work
Will not be done,
Till grief itself
Dies, in childbirth –
Its progeny hope's glimmer,
Lighting the darkest recess
Of a breaking heart.

About the time that was written (some four months after Mary had died) I had 'flu very badly, and woke in the small hours to find that I had lost my voice completely. It was the second time this had happened – the first time had been within a few days of Mary's dying, the result of talking for hours on end. It was almost to be expected in those circumstances, and in a different state of mind I might even have welcomed it as a valid excuse for stopping talking altogether, for the time being.

If that thought had been in even the back of my mind, it was to vanish altogether with the disappearance of my voice. As I tried to speak, another altogether different kind of panic struck me – totally unanticipated – as it came to me that this was what Mary had had to put up with during the last few weeks of her life, yet with no sign even of frustration, let alone panic. It was another of those 'unacknowledged pains', buried deep in my unconscious, and erupting with terrifying power as I identified with Mary's plight, in the midst of my own.

That second time it happened, when I had 'flu, was to be the most horrendous manifestation I had ever experienced of the eruptive power which lies beneath a repressed and undigested emotion. Everything conspired to make it so: the fact that it happened in the small hours, when life is at its lowest ebb; that I was on my own, and worse still, at such an hour unable to call on any human help, even on the telephone. Who could I ring up at three in the morning, to whisper as best I could that 'flu had caused me to lose my voice, and that I was in a state of panic in consequence? How to explain, at such a time of night, the dread which had been rammed into the deep hold of my mind, and had had the hatches battened down on it?

For four hours, and keeping as still as possible, I repeated over and over and over in my mind, hundreds of times, a little 'dart prayer' of Julian of Norwich, which, fortunately for me, I had come across a few months earlier, and had made use of, in calmer waters: "God, of your goodness, give me yourself, for you are enough for me".

It was the thought, "you are enough", that I clung to so desperately until the dawn, when I felt that I could in good conscience ring someone up.

After the 'flu, insomnia (which had never been far away) and a month on Temazipam, prescribed by a junior doctor. The drug was little or no use against the effects of the depression left behind by the 'flu, which was almost the last straw, but it yielded an hour or two of fitful unconsciousness each night, desperately needed to separate one day from the next. Without that brief respite from my own company, I felt I would go under altogether.

At the end of the month I went to renew the prescription, and happened upon the senior partner this time.

"You know, Temazipam is seriously addictive," he said, adding immediately, "You ought to get off it as quickly as possible."

"Then don't give me the prescription. I'll have to find a way of doing without it, won't I?" I responded.

We were almost into December, and the run-up to Christmas. Everything was beginning to pile up now, with a speed and an inexorability which was terrifying. Awful though it is to admit, even without the complications of the 'flu and insomnia I had been dreading this first Christmas without Mary. I believe that is a common experience in bereavement. There were the cards, too – we usually sent over a hundred of them – and the presents for family and friends. Such was the malaise of spirit that had come upon me so catastrophically, that if I could have done, I would have wiped Christmas off the calendar for 1988.

The most immediate problem was making up my mind about going to Rosemary in Germany for the holiday period. In the state I was in, boarding a plane for Stuttgart felt as remotely possible as boarding a spacecraft for the Moon. Moreover, doing without Temazipam was proving to be easier said than done, and virtually sleepless nights were not making decision-taking any easier. Nevertheless, the decision was made to go to Germany, aided and abetted by the community nursing sister who had been involved in getting Mary into hospital in June, and who had held a watching brief over me ever since Mary had died. How important that lifeline was at that time, and how much more important than whole bottlesful of Temazipam!

For a few days it seemed that the air had cleared a little, though the grim struggle for sleep went on. Then, suddenly, something snapped. A desperately tense day was followed by an equally desperate night, and the next day can only be described as a descent into hell. I remember saying to a friend who witnessed what was happening that I would not have dreamed of wishing the experience upon even my worst enemy. One speaks of jangled nerves, but what was happening that day felt as though every negative emotion I had ever had was battering at my consciousness simultaneously. It was emotional bedlam.

I can but record the bare facts of what happened during the next 48 hours, and leave them to speak for themselves, how they will.

Somehow or other, I got myself to a homeopathic doctor in the city, of whom I had heard good reports, who, having listened for the better part of an hour to some account of the parlous state I was in, thought quietly for several minutes, then gave me a single pellet, there and then, with two more, to be taken in the next two days. I was warned that, in accordance with the principles of homeopathic medicine, I would probably feel worse before I felt better. I did – much worse. At the same time a doctor friend of the orthodox ilk said I must get some sleep of some sort, and recommended that I took Temazipam again, at least for one night. Remember – I had recently been taking Temazipam for a whole month with near disastrous effects, so that what happened next cannot possibly be attributed to that single extra capsule I took that night. I did sleep, not particularly well, nor particularly badly, but what I experienced on waking the next morning can only be described as near-miraculous. Gone altogether was the fierce jangle of the emotional clamour of the day before, and in its place peace, the peace of a summer's day following a violent thunderstorm. I remember saying to the homeopathic doctor that I felt like a snake who had shed its skin, and back came the reply at once, that that was what she had been hoping and expecting to hear me say.

I continued with the treatment for another ten days, and since that time, though there have been many emotional upheavals on the road back to a full life, there has never been anything to compare with the hell of those two days in November 1988.

As a scientist I know all the arguments purporting to prove that homeopathy just cannot work, and that at best it relies on the placebo effect for its successes; but in point of fact my most spectacular experience of it was in the face of my own scepticism and a near-total despair that there was anything left in this world which could be of any help to me at all. Perhaps all our orthodoxies, religious and scientific alike, need to be tested to destruction, from time to time.

Christmas in Germany brought its own problems, some of them anticipated, some not.

There was the matter of sheer distance, which I could well have anticipated from a previous experience in 1981, when motoring to the Isle of Mull with friends, for a painting holiday. We started at six in the morning, Mary having taken up residence in the Holiday Home the evening before. We were due to catch a ferry in the early evening at Oban, nearly 500 miles north. We took the driving in turn, two hours at a stretch, stopping only briefly for meals. As we pressed on, hour after hour after hour, I had a strange, steadily growing, and ever more disturbing feeling that I was getting too far away from Mary – that she was passing out of reach. It had something to do with the ceaseless sound of the engine, and the endless motion of the countryside from being ahead of us to being behind us, to put more and more distance between Mary and me.

Mary's physical dependence on me – and I must emphasise physical dependence – had much in common with the physical dependence of a child on its mother; and my feelings, too, that day, must have had much in common with those of a mother being forcibly taken away from her child. And as we climbed Shap Fell, and approached the Scottish border, I had what was my first taste of panic on Mary's behalf, all those years ago. I was sitting in the back of the car at the time, having just completed my stint of driving, when, suddenly, I felt I could go no further – that I must get out of the car there and then, and go back home. I remember having to fight off the feeling – of wanting to say to my friends, "Stop the car! You must go on without me."

Re-living that experience, I realise now that I was already beginning to have an identity problem as early as 1981, the boundaries between Mary's life and my own already becoming blurred; but it went unrecognised, and became yet another of those

> Unacknowledged pains
> Deep buried
> By the wayside
> Of our journey
> Through those stricken years,

only to erupt again with such ferocity, after Mary had died.

So too it was, in Germany, though the feeling did stop short of panic. But the sense of having travelled too far from Mary (though quite irrational, for she was dead now) was almost as acute as it had been in 1981.

The sense of isolation was increased in a quite unanticipated manner, too. In one's own country one is linked with everyone around one by the mother tongue, enjoying the subconscious experience of belonging, of being the visible part of one's roots buried below, in one's native 'soil'. But, in Rosemary's home, as the usual stream of Christmas visitors came and went, my tourist German, sufficient to get me by in a shop, or when asking for the bus station, was quite inadequate to enable me to feel part of the festivities, as the conversation ebbed and flowed over the crumbling Stolle, and I began to feel more and more excluded from the company. Rosemary, of course, could do nothing about it: the visitors were more often than not casual ones, who spoke little or no English.

It got worse, with the sense that the family was scattered, some of it on holiday in France, some of it in Germany, and some of it still back in England, with Mary no longer amongst us, with, so to say, her brood about her. I began to feel that I would have to cut my visit short, and go home: if one was to be lonely, better to be lonely among familiar things. Instead, however, I went out and used what little German I had to buy a short-wave radio, so that I could listen, almost like one of the hostages, to the BBC World Service.

It was January 2nd, and by mere serendipity (was it merely that?) almost the first thing I heard was a five-minute New Year's religious broadcast. The speaker read a passage from *The Shaking of the Foundations*, by the American existential theologian, Paul Tillich. I had the book at home, but hadn't looked at it in years.

Nothing is more surprising than the rise of the new within ourselves. We do not foresee or observe its growth. We do not try to produce it by the strength of our will, by the power of our emotion, or by the clarity of our intellect. On the contrary, we feel that by trying to produce it we prevent its coming. By trying, we would produce the old in the power of the old, but not the new in the power of the new. The new being is born in us, just when we least believe in it. It appears in remote corners of our souls which we have neglected for a long time. It opens up deep levels of our personality which had been shut out by old decisions and old exclusions. It shows a way where there was no way before. It liberates us from the tragedy of having to decide and having to exclude, because it is given before any decision. Suddenly we notice it within us! The new which we sought and longed for comes to us in the moment in which we lose hope of ever finding it... It appears when and where it chooses. We cannot force it, and we cannot calculate it. Readiness is the only condition for it; and readiness means that the former things have become old and that they are driving us into the destruction of our souls just when we are trying most to save what we think can be saved of the old.

I lapped up the words like a thirsty dog who had come upon a stream of clear mountain water after a long and arid trek: "The new being is born in us, just when we least believe in it ... It shows a way where there was no way before ... The new which we sought and longed for comes to us in the moment in which we lose hope of ever finding it ... Readiness is the only condition ... and readiness means that the former things have become old and that they are driving us to the destruction of our souls just when we are trying most to save what we think can be saved from the old...."

That, surely, meant that I was as ready as anyone could be. As I thought about it a deep and wide and blessed assurance flooded over me – that this was the truth for me, the truth which, so to say, had been knocking at the door for so long, trying to get me simply to open to it. There was no clutching at straws, nothing of that feeling that here at least and at last was a faint flicker of truth which, if I clung to it hard enough, might stay, and perhaps even grow. No, there was nothing partial about the truth the words were presenting, it was truth seen in the broad, as though scales had suddenly fallen from my eyes. It was like someone switching on the light in a darkened room – there it all was, an orderly place, instead of the chaos that I had been imagining. It was truth 'in the round' – truth that was, as I like to put it, completely 'self-validating'.

I could hardly wait to get home. I knew that apart from *The Shaking of the Foundations* there were at least three other books by Paul Tillich, waiting on my shelves. Even their titles spoke volumes! – *The New Being, The Eternal Now*, and *The Courage To Be*. I began to devour them, marking whole passages in them, page after page, reading them again and again, even adding them to my library of micro-cassettes, so that I could listen to them on a bus, or a country walk. They became dog-eared, and *The Shaking of the Foundations*, (appropriately enough, in a way) finally fell to pieces, and had to be held together after that with rubber bands.

Was it all over then? – this herculean struggle for peace of mind and spirit, and the beginning of new life and new being? According to Gabriel Marcel, "It is never a simple return to the status quo, a simple return to our being, it is that and much more ... an undreamed-of promotion, a transfiguration." Was this it, then?

There was always that possibility, I suppose. But, with Paul Tillich, I was to discover that "the new ... must break the power of the old, not only in reality, but in our memory; and one is not possible without the other." From then on there were to be increasingly long passages through calm waters; and never again was the patch of blue in the storm sky to appear quite so small, or the blackness under the trees quite so impenetrable. But memory, with its sombre brood – of pain, and never-ending sense of loss, of nostalgia, ever mingled with regret – was to remain for long a stumbling block.

There are times, too – and perhaps always will be – when my "courage to be", no match for Mary's anyway, forsakes me still – with

Each day
A lifetime:

Each waking
A birth,
With its fierce pang
For the lost womb
Of the night,
Its first breath
Deep-drawn in protest
At the burgeoning of day;

Each morning
A childhood,
Deprived of its
Innocent obliviousness
Of Man's mortality;

High noon
A middle age
Of unfulfilled
Intentions
Failing to survive
The close scrutiny
Of day;

Each afternoon
A retirement, forfeit
To a frantic foraging
For the mislaid meaning
Of the past and hope
With which to face
A boding future;

Each evening
An old age
Graced,
Surprisingly enough,
By a brief acceptance
Of things as they are;

And night
A return
To the darkness
Of unknowing.

Earlier, much earlier in these pages, there was mention of a little talk I had heard on the radio at Christmastide, several years ago. Entitled *A Wink of Heaven*, it seemed to me to embody the very heart of the Christian message.

Having spoken of how uncertain life can be and more often than not is, in the big issues as well as the small, the speaker went on to ask, "What has all this talk of uncertainty to do with Christmas Day?" He continued:

> The birth of Christ was foretold centuries earlier, and Christians say it was divinely planned before the beginning of time. And yet, when it happened, it could not have been more unrehearsed: he was born into a makeshift set-up amid people who were simply improvising as they went along.... If God was giving Himself to humanity in this child, then he was surrendering himself to uncertainty; and this is the 'wink of heaven', this is the 'whisper' that Christmas brings us – that God, in his relationship with this world, has always surrendered Himself to uncertainty. "'Emmanuel' – 'God with us' – that is the name the prophet gave to the child who was to be born. 'God with us' in all the accidental chanciness and the moral uncertainties of this life. He won't give you a nicely-painted signpost... He will give you Himself. God doesn't make things happen – he takes what has happened and he says 'What shall we make of this?'"

Yes – "God with us" in the accidental chanciness of the hurricane and the flood, the heart attack and the stroke. He doesn't make any of these things happen, but he is there, alongside us, sharing the uncertainty and the agony – surely 'the one thing needful' for us to know.

It was TS Eliot who, in *Murder in the Cathedral*, had Thomas à Becket say, as he was about to meet his assassins, "I have had a tremor of bliss, a wink of heaven, a whisper...."

Was that the 'whisper' that Mary had heard, and which, all along, had been the source of her sort of courage?

The Poems

You saw me first tonight –
And waved!
And made a space for me,
A place for me,
Beside you,
On the bed.

Right from the start
We talked –
Oh, how we talked! –
You plainly,
So plainly, at first;
And after,
In that little burble
Interspersed
With laughter;
For tonight what matter
That meanings sometimes went astray
In wordless chatter?

What matter?
We met! –
Oh, how we met! –
In a fourth dimension –
Not of Einstein's time,
But freed
Of its constraint
And tension –
Where future
Had no past,
And past no future:
And the present moment,
Fleeting no longer,
Became
The Eternal Now –
The place
Of all
True meeting.

Slow steps
On familiar ground,
With carpet's edge
A dangerous ledge,
And single stair
A precipice,
Fraught
With grave peril:
The mountaineer
In all his strength,
Roped
To stalwart colleagues,
With the blue sky
And the towering peaks
Above
To challenge him,
Knows nothing
Of your sort of courage;
His risk
Seems small,
And his objective
Near,
Compared with yours,
A few feet away;
As,
Scorning help,
With walking frame
And caliper
You move,
Step by step,
Precariously,
Alone in your weakness
Towards
The fireside chair.

The year wears on –
The magic mists appear,
Casting their immemorial spell;
And leaves,
Fresh green when you were well,
Are turning brown, then red,
And, twisting in the chill wind, fall
As dead –
Trees shedding
Their sad confetti.

Daily, the artist sun,
With prodigal palette,
Paints cosmic canvases;
And, night by night,
The stark stars,
Piercing the canopy of evening,
Stave off, still,
The gathering dark.

And birds, on branch and eave,
Incredulously yet sing,
To catch my spirit
Off-guard,
And evoke
The fierce pang
Of remembered joy –
Joy that I scarce now
Dare contemplate.

Joy is no joy
That needs to state its terms,
And so deny its own true nature –
Which
Of such substance is,
That neither time
Nor chance,
Nor circumstance
Erodes –
Or ever can.

Too easy it was,
By far,
To take you for granted
When you were well:
All too easy
To be preoccupied
With trivia –
To open the door
And peck you with a kiss
And say,
Straightway,
"Do you know
What so-and-so did
Today?"
Too easy
To but half-listen,
And never to stop
And wonder
At the music of your voice;
To let pass,
Unsung,
Your grace of movement,
The marvellous coordination
Of foot with foot,
Which we call
Walking –
Too easy,
All too easy,
So.

Menus on the tables,
Places neatly laid –
Sparkling glasses
Waiting to be filled –
Chairs disposed
Invitingly;
And, over all,
The soft light
Of the table lamps,
Casting their benedictory air.

I thought of the time –
Oh, so little time ago! –
When I took you out
To dine:
We sat in the sixteenth-century bay,
Overhanging the busy street,
As, Elizabethan-gay,
We laughed,
And ate,
And studied the passers-by.
And the toast was
"To us!",
As we raised the wine,
And your right hand
Held the glass –
Oh, God! –
Your right hand
Held the glass.

Pull up the chairs!
Poke up the fire!
And curl up,
Cosily!
For this week's
Colour Supplement
Invites us
To choose
Where we might go –
To escape
The winter
Within.

And let the chatter
Be loud enough
That the sound
Of the moan
In the wind
May be drowned.
Turn on the light!
Draw curtains tight!
(Yes! turn on
Sweet music, too)
And we'll play a game
Of make-pretend
That there is no darkness
Outside:
Better to bask
In fluorescent tube's light
Than risk
An encounter
With God,
In the night.

"Bloody bad luck,"
He said,
As he drove from the fifteenth tee,
But it was not of his drive
That he spoke,
But of me.
(His ball went into the rough.)

> "Yes –
> His wife –
> It happened in June,
> And we've hardly seen him since;
> They despaired of her life
> At the time –
> Even now she can't be left."
> (They searched for the little white ball,
> Which, of course, was all in all –
> 'Three off the tee'
> It would otherwise be.)
> "Damned bad luck –
> Just think –
> He's probably washing up!"
> (I was).
> "Poor bloody bod,
> Perhaps
> He's even
> Praying to God."
> (That also was true.)

They found the ball
(And another one, too),
And he chopped it out
With his Nine.
"We might save the hole,"
(His partner said)
"If the next one
Finds the green –
Yes, it's damned bad luck
When a chap has to chuck
His golf."

> By the time they had reached
> The Nineteenth,
> The washing-up was done,
> And my belov'd was up and dressed,
> And settled in her chair;
> And had started to practise
> To write her name
> With a hand that still rebelled,
> As they downed their beers,
> And swallowed their fears
> That life might not be
> Always
> A game.

Early morning
Gives no warning
Of a sunset
Less than eternity away:
No need to plan the day.

Mid-morning
Is refreshment time –
Let's take a breather
From our play
(The sunshine has surely come to stay!)

High noon,
And native powers
Intoxicate
With the sense
That the choice is ours:
There is nothing we could not do
If we wanted to –
But we don't.
By afternoon
The shadow
Of a doubt
Appears:
The sun seems not quite so high
(Could it be that it threatens
To set –
And that in a finite time?)

Late afternoon,
And a nip in the air –
Better to have a care –
There is no doubt now
That the night exists,
And the light is getting low.

But –
Could it be
That sun's dying glow
Yet symbols
A promise,
Born of diminishment
And fulfilled
At day's end?

Love has a currency
    All its own:
Its smallest denomination
Is of inestimable worth –
Yet it is theft-proof,
And thus needs no protection.
       Minted freely,
        It creates no fear of inflation –
        In fact, it reverses
        All the usual rules.

Thus, unless it is counterfeit,
Its investment
Seeks no return;
And income actually increases
With expenditure.
        Its nature is always to be
        A gift –
        It cannot therefore be earned,
        Or claimed as any kind of recompense
        Or reward;
        And, when returned,
        It needs to be immediately reinvested;
        For the attempt to hoard it
        Leads to bankruptcy.

It defies
Drawing up a balance sheet,
For it cannot be enumerated;
And any attempt
To put a price on it
Renders it worthless.
It is always available on demand,
And requires no security:
Indeed,
It may take the form
Of a blank cheque,
With the consequences
Willingly accepted;
For counting the cost
Is foreign to it.
        It is exchangeable
        The world over,
        But such exchange
        Must always be
        Person to person:
        No broker
        Can have dealings in it
        To achieve a cheap gain.

It can be taxed
To the limit,
Yet emerge
With enhanced reserves:
It is the only currency
Adequate to meet the cost
Of living.

The world goes by:
Young lovers kiss
In the streets;
And ageing couples
Saunter,
Scanning the windows
For bargains
In tomorrow's sales;
Old people sit,
Slightly apart,
On the seats;
And young bloods
Thunder past
Astride their machines,
Thirsting for trouble,
Oblivious, all,
Of the miracle
Of arms
And legs,
And simple conversation.

Now you are coming home,
My love –
Home to us all!
Yet, were truth better served
To say that home
Is coming back to us –
For you are home!
Bricks and mortar
Have ever been
Merely the place
For you to be
What you are:
Wife,
Mother,
Friend of all!
So!
Sing bricks!
Sing mortar!
And sing, my darling daughter!
Rejoice, my sons!
For home is coming back
To each and all
Of us.

Not to get used
To the sound of your foot
Dragging reluctantly
Across the floor
Behind your walking frame,
Which you manoeuvre
Like an unwilling mule
You are desperately trying
To tame;

> Not to get used
> To the sight of your face,
> Frustration-fraught,
> As you strive for the word
> That is pikestaff-plain
> To your inner eye –
> But you struggle to say
> In vain;

Not to get used
To the clutch of your hand
On my arm
As we dare the two steps
To the garden below –
A journey whose hazards
You, only, can know;

> Not to get used
> To the thought
> That once was a time
> When foot followed foot
> In so graceful
> A walk,
> And word followed word
> In a torrent
> Of talk,
> And arm tucked in arm
> Just for love
> Not support;

God!
Not to get used
To these things,
I say –
Not to get used to them, God,
I pray...

Let me
At least take comfort
From my tears –
That there is yet left
Enough of me
To weep,
Not simply, now, for loss of you,
But for a myriad
Unacknowledged pains
Deep buried
By the wayside
Of our journey
Through those stricken years.

"I weep,
Therefore I am" –
Thus do I reassure myself
That desolation
Has not laid final waste
To me;
Yet
On that journey
Did I, like those
In heat of battle smitten,
Soldier on,
Unaware
That when the strife was at an end
I would have mortal wounds
To tend.

Weep then,
Scan the bleak landscape
Of those fraught, fateful years,
Drink the full draught
Of unassimilated pain,
And the then unshed,
Countless tears.

Many said
That it was over now;
Others, that I should be thankful;
A few (I fear) that it was simply
God's will that had been done,
(Like the hurricane last year) –
But I knew the life, which,
In my heart,
Had only just begun.

Death gave it birth: your passing
The cosmic contraction
That propelled me
On the headfirst journey
Through the tortuous tunnel
Of fierce disbelief –
With pain beyond thought –
Into a future
Furnished
With an empty chair,
An empty bed,
Coats still hanging, ready,
In the hall;
Your place at table vacant,
Meal on meal.

Morning upon morning,
Listless and leaden-eyed
I lie,
Hoping the world
Will pass me by.
What chance of that? –
The harsh light of reality
Leaves no margin
For the re-interpretation
Of events;
Better to weep my way
Into the crevices
Of yet another day –
Others, perchance,
Will neither find
Nor even seek me
There.

But –
Tread warily;
At every twist and turn
Of time
And space
There lies in wait
Some devastating evocation
Of the past –
Beyond tears:
From a paper scrap,

With frail words
Traced by that rebellious hand,
To your first caliper, lurking
In the dark depths
Of a wardrobe
Where I sought
A long-lost pair of shoes.
(God alone knows
The volumes spoken
By a piece of bent iron
Fitted with a leather thong
And metal peg –
The vision, too,
That it evoked
Of you,
With your strapped leg
And walking frame,
And those first faltering steps –
God, indeed, alone knows
The courage that you showed.)

Beyond tears, yes,
But weep noneless;
Grief's work
Will not be done,
Till grief itself
Dies, in childbirth –
Its progeny hope's glimmer,
Lighting the darkest recess
Of a breaking heart.

Each day
A lifetime:

Each waking
A birth,
With its fierce pang
For the lost womb
Of the night,
Its first breath
Deep-drawn in protest
At the burgeoning of day;

Each morning
A childhood,
Deprived of its
Innocent obliviousness
Of Man's mortality;

High noon
A middle age
Of unfulfilled
Intentions
Failing to survive
The close scrutiny
Of day;

Each afternoon
A retirement, forfeit
To a frantic foraging
For the mislaid meaning
Of the past and hope
With which to face
A boding future;

Each evening
An old age
Graced,
Surprisingly enough,
By a brief acceptance
Of things as they are;

And night
A return
To the darkness
Of unknowing.

List of Addresses

The Stroke Association
CHSA House
Whitecross Street
London
EC1Y 8JJ
0171 490 7999

**National Association of
  Bereavement Services**
20 Norton Folgate
London
E1 6DB
0171 241 1080

Cruse – Bereavement Care
Cruse House
126 Sheen Road
Richmond
Surrey
TW9 1UR
Bereavement Line: 0181 332 7227

Carers National Association
29 Chilworth Mews
London
W2 3RG
0171 490 8898

**British Association for Service
  to the Elderly**
119 Hassell Street
Newcastle-under-Lyme
Staffs ST5 1AX
01782 661033